STARVI CANCER AND WIN THE FIGHT!

Complete Guide to Medical Breakthroughs in Cancer Therapy that Will Give You Upper Hand in Your Battle With Cancer

are mentioned are done without written consent and can in no way be considered an endorsement from the trademark holder.

TABLE OF CONTENTS.

DESCRIPTION

Learn How to Turn Your Body into Cancer-Hostile Environment That Will Starve the Cancer and Kill it for Good

For many years, scientists have been trying to stop cancer by blocking nutrients from reaching tumor cells, effectively robbing tumor cells of the food required to expand and proliferate. These attempts were in vain because cancer cells are agile, and they depend on multiple contingency routes to continue their expansion.

The scientists have manipulated specific weak points in the metabolism of cancer cells, causing tumor cells to expose backup fuel supply routes on which they rely when this vulnerability is disrupted.

Are you fighting a battle with cancer? Would you like to gain the upper hand and acquire tools to turn your body into a cancer-hostile environment?

Your battle is not an easy one, dear reader. But the information is your greatest weapon. You need to inform yourself on how does cancer work, how does it "eat, breathes, and lives," and that's precisely what this book offers.

This is not some "dieting" guide that will tell you to eat this and to stop eating that without any proof. This book contains only scientifically backed claims that are proven to work!

Here is what this book can offer you:

- All about the cancer – how it works, how it eats, how it grows

- Everything you need to know about starving a cancer

- Foods that are proven to have anti-cancer properties

- In-depth explanation of synergistic cancer starvation therapy – antiangiogenesis combined with chemotherapy, gene therapy, or phototherapy

- Everything about VDAs based cancer starvation therapy

- And much more!

If you want to successfully fight off the cancer, this book will give you the means and knowledge to do so. It's up to you what you will use in the battle. Stay strong, and remember, you are not alone in this fight.

INTRODUCTIONS

For decades, scientists have been trying to stop cancer by blocking nutrients from reaching tumor cells, effectively robbing tumor cells from the food required to expand and proliferate. These attempts have also been frustrated that cancer cells are nimble, depending on multiple contingency routes to continue to expand.

Researchers have manipulated a specific weak point in the metabolism of cancer cells, causing tumor cells to expose backup fuel supply routes on which they rely when this vulnerability is disrupted. Mapping these secondary pathways, researchers have also established drugs that block them. A major clinical study of cancer patients is currently being prepared to test this therapeutic approach.

Like a healthy cell, a sarcoma cell depends on external supplies of arginine, an essential building block of proteins. Remove environmental arginine and the cell must initiate a cycle called autophagy, or "self-eating," to live. A second attack on the survival mechanism, then destroys the cells Studying human cancer cells and the mice injected with patient tumor samples, the researchers prove that a double strike — the elimination of the weak point and one of the tumor cells 'replacement pathways — is effective against several hard-to-treat cancers. While found in several forms of cancer, the weak point is especially prominent in sarcomas — rare skin, muscle, bone, cartilage, and connective tissue cancers, doctors treat sarcomas mainly with conventional surgery, radiation and chemotherapy, although these therapies are sometimes not successful.

It is known that this metabolic deficiency is found in 90% of sarcomas Healthy cells may not have this flaw. We have been attempting to establish a treatment that takes advantage of the metabolic deficiency so, ideally, it can only treat the tumor. Essentially, the mutation helps one to compel the tumor cells to die. "In order to expand and proliferate, the tumor cells must have simple building materials. The work approach is focused on the assumption that the overwhelming majority of sarcomas have missed the capacity to produce their own arginine, a protein building block that cells use to create more of themselves. In the absence of this capacity, the cells will extract arginine from the external area. The stock of arginine in the blood is sufficient, and the cancer cells have little trouble scavenging it. But removing the environmental supply of arginine and cells is a issue.

"If we use a medication to deplete arginine in the blood, the cancer cells fear as they have depleted their fuel source," Van Tine said. "Now they're rewiring to continue and live. For this research, we used this rewiring to classify medications that block secondary pathways. "Like other cancer treatments, the loss of arginine in the blood does not impact healthy cells. Healthy cells do not depend on foreign sources of arginine since they may not have a metabolic deficiency in the cancer. We tend to produce their own arginine, but there is no mediated malnutrition in regular cells even though there is no arginine in the blood. This technique is focused on the tumor's properties — specifically, it shuts down tumor metabolism and nothing else.

Unable to produce or receive external arginine, the fuel supply routes of the tumor cells are pushed inward. Cells may continue to metabolize their internal supply of arginine in a cycle called autophagy or self-eating. In the case of sarcomas, it delays or delays down the development of cancer but does not destroy the cell. Throughout this phase, tumor cells seem to be buying time to rediscover another internal work-around.

"Cancer doesn't disappear because you interrupt the primary fuel source," Van Tine said. "Because of this, it transforms all these roads to redemption. Within this article, we established the mechanisms of salvage. And we found that when you poison them, you destroy the cells, too. Our research has shown that tumors are gradually diminishing in these conditions. It is the first time that tumors have been shown to reduce utilizing only metabolic medications with no other anti-cancer approaches.

The arginine-depleting medication is now in clinical studies evaluating its protection with efficacy against kidney, lung, pancreatic, breast and other cancers. But, to date, it has been unlikely to succeed as it has triggered the regeneration mechanisms that enable cancer growth to begin. Researchers also proposed that the medication can still be a critical mitochondrial treatment for cancer as long as it is used in conjunction with other medications targeting replacement pathways.

If cancer cells with this metabolic deficiency are depleted of environmental arginine, they are required to switch from a glucose-burning mechanism to a mechanism that consumes another fuel called glutamine. Researchers also demonstrated that the application of a glutamine receptor to the arginine-depleting product is toxic to the cells. Eliminating arginine from the blood often re-wires serine biology, another backup power, and incorporating serine inhibitors often triggers cell death.

This technique may be extended outside uncommon sarcoma tumors, since the metabolic disorder is also found in many cancers, including other forms of breast, colon, lung, brain, and bone tumors, the researchers said. The latest research provides evidence demonstrating specific anti-tumor responses in cell lines of both forms of cancer.

Both medications used in the research are now currently licensed by the U.S. Health and Medication Treatment for various diseases or in current clinical studies on cancer medications.

Calorie restriction (CR) reduces malnutrition and has anticancer activity in multiple preclinical models. CR is gradually being extended to human cancer as a sensitizing technique before chemotherapy regimens. Although the beneficial effects of CR are generally recognized, the processes by which CR influences tumor growth are not well known. In several cell types, CR and other nutritional stress may cause autophagy, which offers energy and metabolic substrates that are vital to survival. We believed that reducing the supply of extracellular and intracellular substrate by combining CR with autophagy inhibition would suppress tumor growth more efficiently than either drug alone.

Results: The 30 per cent CR diet opposed to control diet in nude mice resulted in substantial reductions in body weight, blood glucose, cortisol, cortisol-like growth factor 1 and leptin rates at the same period as elevated adiponectin rates.

Metabolic analyzes of CR-fed, compared to control-fed, nude mice revealed substantial reductions in circulating glucose and amino acids and large rises in ketones, suggesting a change to fat metabolism.

In a nude mouse xenograft model involving H-RasG12V-transformed immortal kid mouse renal epithelial cells with (Atg5+/+) and without (Atg5-/-) autophagic ability, the CR diet significantly reduced tumor development. Tumor formation and growth was highest for Atg5+/+ tumors in control-fed mice, moderate for both Atg5+/+ tumors in CR-fed mice and Atg5-/-tumours in control-fed mice, and lowest for Atg5-/-tumours in CR mice. In Atg5+/+ tumors, autophagic flux was increased in CR-fed relative to control-fed mice, indicating that the pro-survival effects of autophagic induction that counteract the tumor suppression effects of CR. Conclusions: Combined restriction of extracellular (via CR) and intracellular (via autophagy inhibition) energy sources and nutrients inhibits Ras-driven tumor development more efficiently than either CR or autophagy deficiency alone. Interventions addressing both systemic energy balance and tumor-cell intestinal autophagy can reflect a new anticancer strategy.

CHAPTER ONE
WHAT IS CANCER

Cancer is the term assigned to the group of diseases connected to it. In both forms of cancer, certain cells of the body tend to differentiate without stopping and spread to neighboring tissues.

Cancer may begin virtually anywhere in the human body, which is made up of billions of cells. Normally, human cells expand and split in order to create new cells when the body requires them. As cells grow old or become injured, they die, and new cells take their place.

Nonetheless, this organized mechanism breaks down as cancer arises. When cells are more and more dysfunctional, old or weakened cells live until they die, and new cells develop when they are not required. Such extra cells may grow without stopping and can develop tumors called tumors.

Most cancers develop solid tumors, which are tissue masses. Blood cancers, such as leukemia, usually do not develop solid tumors.

Cancer tumors are malignant, which means they can grow to or enter surrounding tissues. In fact, as such tumors develop, certain cancer cells can break down and migrate to distant parts of the body via the blood or lymph system, creating new tumors far from the original tumor.

Unlike malignant tumors, benign cancers may not grow to or attack surrounding tissues. Nevertheless, benign tumors can often be very big. Normally, they do not grow again after extracted, though malignant tumors often do. Like other benign cancers in many areas of the body, benign brain tumors may be life threatening.

Differences between Cancer Cells and Normal Cells

Cancer cells vary in several respects from regular cells that cause them to develop out of control and become invasive. An essential distinction is that cancer cells are less advanced than regular cells. This is, although regular cells develop into very distinct cell forms with different roles, cancer cells do not. It is one explanation that, unlike regular cells, cancer cells tend to grow without halting.

In fact, cancer cells are able to disregard signs that usually warn cells to avoid dividing or start a cycle known as programmed cell death, or apoptosis that the body uses to get rid of unneeded cells.

Cancer cells may affect normal cells, proteins, and blood vessels that surround and support the tumor — an region known as the microenvironment. For example, cancer cells may stimulate neighboring normal cells to create blood vessels that provide oxygen and nutrients to tumors that they need to expand. Such blood vessels also absorb tumor waste materials.

Cancer cells are most frequently able to escape the immune system, the network of muscles, tissues, and specialist cells that defend the body against diseases and other disorders. While the immune system usually destroys weakened or dysfunctional cells from the body, certain cancer cells are able to escape from the immune system.

Tumors can also use the immune system to remain alive and develop. Of example, with the aid of some immune system cells that usually inhibit a uncontrolled immune reaction, cancer cells may potentially block the immune system from destroying cancer cells.

Fundamentals of Cancer

In regular cells, tumor suppression genes inhibit cancer by reducing or halting cell development. DNA changes that inactivate tumor suppressor genes can lead to unregulated cell growth and cancer.

Inside the tumor, cancer cells are covered by a number of immune cells, fibroblasts, proteins, and blood vessels — what is recognized as the microenvironment of the tumor. Cancer cells can influence the microenvironment, which in effect may impact the development and spread of cancer.

Immune system cells can detect and destroy cancer cells. But certain cancer cells may resist or inhibit an attack from occurring. Many cancer therapies can enable the immune system to better recognize and destroy cancer cells.

Each person's cancer has a particular mix of genetic variations. Relevant genetic variations can render a individual more or less likely to react to certain treatments.

Genetic alterations that induce cancer can be hereditary or can result from other reactions to the climate. Genetic variations can often arise due to errors that arise when cells split.

Much of the time, cancer-causing genetic variations occur gradually as a individual ages, contributing to a higher chance of cancer later in life.

Cancer cells may split free from the initial tumor and migrate through the blood or lymph system to distant sites in the body, leaving the vessels to create new tumors. It's also metastases.

Cancer is a cancer triggered when cells grow uncontrollably and spread to neighboring tissues.

Cancer is triggered by Genetic modifications. Many cancer-causing Genetic modifications arise in Genetic pieces called chromosomes. These variations are often referred to as genetic changes.

A shift in DNA may trigger the genes involved in normal cell growth to become oncogenes. Unlike regular genes, oncogenes can not be switched off, which induces unregulated cell development.

Within normal cells, tumor suppression genes inhibit cancer by preventing or halting cell development. DNA changes that inactivate tumor suppressor genes can lead to unregulated cell growth and cancer.

Inside the tumor, cancer cells are covered by a number of immune cells, fibroblasts, proteins, and blood vessels — what is recognized as the microenvironment of the tumor. Cancer cells can influence the microenvironment, which in effect may impact the development and spread of cancer.

Immune system cells can detect and destroy cancer cells. But certain cancer cells may resist or inhibit an attack from occurring. Many cancer therapies can enable the immune system to better recognize and destroy cancer cells.

Each person's cancer has a particular mix of genetic variations. Relevant genetic variations can render a individual more or less likely to react to certain treatments.

Genetic alterations that induce cancer can be hereditary or can result from other reactions to the climate. Genetic variations can often arise due to errors that arise when cells split.

Much of the time, cancer- genetic variations occur gradually as a individual ages, contributing to a higher chance of cancer later in life.

Cancer cells may split free from the initial tumor and migrate through the blood or lymph system to distant sites in the body, leaving the vessels to create new tumors. It's also metastases.

How Cancer Occurs

Cancer is induced by such gene modifications, the essential physical units of inheritance. Genes are contained in large stretches of closely compressed DNA labeled chromosomes.

Cancer is a genetic disease — that is, it is triggered by gene changes that regulate how our cells work, particularly how they develop and divide.

Genetic variations that cause cancer can be inherited by our ancestors. These can often arise during a person's lifespan as a consequence of mistakes that develop when cells differentiate or as a consequence of DNA damage induced by other reactions to the environment. Cancer-causing occupational pollutants include things such as cigarette smoking additives and heat, such as ultraviolet sunlight. Each person's cancer has a particular mix of genetic variations. If cancer continues to evolve, there will be further improvements. Multiple cells can have specific genetic variations often inside the same tumor.

By addition, cancer cells contain more genetic variations than regular cells, such as DNA mutations. Many of these modifications may have little to do with cancer; they may be the product rather than the source of cancer.

"Drivers" of Cancer

Genetic alterations that lead to cancer appear to influence three major groups of genes — proto-oncogenes, tumor reduction genes, and DNA repair genes. Such modifications are often referred to as cancer "runners."

Proto-oncogenes are active in the natural development and separation of cells. However, when such genes are altered in other ways or become more active than expected, they may become cancer-causing genes (or oncogenes) that enable cells to develop and thrive if they are not permitted to do so.

Tumor suppressor genes are also active in the regulation of cell development and division. Cells with such defects in tumor suppressor genes can be separated in an unregulated manner.

DNA repair genes are active in the reconstruction of defective

DNA. Mutation cells in these genes continue to produce new mutations in certain genes. Together, these mutations can trigger cancer in the cells.

When scientists also studied more about the genetic alterations that contribute to cancer, they also discovered that certain mutations frequently arise in several forms of cancer. Regardless of that, cancers are often characterized by the kinds of genetic changes that are thought to trigger them, not only about where they grow in the body and how cancer cells appear under the microscope.

What are cancer risk factors and causes

Something that may trigger a regular body cell to grow abnormally possibly may induce cancer. A number of factors can cause cell anomalies and have been related to cancer growth. Many cancer sources remain unexplained, whereas some have environmental or behavioral influences, or can evolve from more than one established source. Others may be developmentally affected by the genetic structure of a individual. Most people grow cancer because of a mixture of these causes.

While it is always challenging or unlikely to determine an event(s) that induces cancer to grow in a single individual, work has provided clinicians with a variety of potential factors that, individually or in combination with other triggers, are likely to be cancer-inducing candidates. The above is a compilation of significant triggers that is not all-inclusive because new factors are regularly introduced because science advances: toxicity to chemical or radioactive compounds:

benzene, asbestos, copper, cadmium, vinyl chloride, benzidine, N-nitrosamines, nicotine or cigarette smoke (contains at least 66 identified possible carcinogenic chemicals that toxins), asbestos, and aflatoxin Ionizing radiation: uranium

Genetics: A variety of common cancers have been related to human genes which are as follows: breast, cervical, colorectal, thyroid, skin which melanoma; actual genes and other specifics remain outside the reach of this general report so that the public is directed to the National Cancer Institute for more information on genetics and cancer.

It is necessary to remember that certain individuals have cancer risk factors and are prone to cancer-causing conditions (e.g. radiation, secondary tobacco smoking, and x-rays) throughout their lifespan, but other individuals will not grow cancer. In fact, many individuals have genes that are related to, but do not grow, cancer. Why? Why? While researchers will not be able to give a reasonable solution to each patient, it is apparent that the higher the volume or degree of cancer-causing materials a person is exposed to, the greater the risk that a person may develop cancer.

In comparison, individuals with hereditary linkages to cancer can not grow it for specific reasons (lack of adequate stimuli to make the genes work). In fact, certain individuals might have an improved immune response that regulates or destroys cells that are or might eventually become cancer cells. There is proof that such nutritional habits may have a major role to play in tandem with the immune system to enable or avoid the survival of cancer cells. It is also impossible to attribute a particular cause of cancer to several people.

Certain contributing factors have also been introduced to the list of things that can raise the likelihood of cancer. In particular, red meat (such as beef, lamb and pork) has been listed as a high-risk cancer-causing agent by the International Organization for Cancer Research; additionally refined meat (salted, grilled, canned and/or cured meat) has been put on the carcinogenic register. Individuals who consume a ton of barbecued meat can often raise their risk due to compounds produced at high temperatures.

Certain loosely specified conditions that can raise the risk of certain cancers include obesity, lack of activity, chronic inflammation, and hormones, including those used for replacement therapy. Certain objects, such as mobile phones, have been thoroughly analyzed. In 2011, the World Health Organization listed low-energy mobile phone exposure as "probably carcinogenic," but this is a very small risk standard that places cell phones at the same risk as coffee and pickled vegetables.

This is impossible to show that a drug may not induce or is not correlated with an elevated risk of cancer. Of starters, certain investigators and not others find antiperspirants to be potentially linked to breast cancer. The NCI's official stance is that "additional work is required to examine this partnership and other variables that could be involved." This unsatisfactory interpretation is provided since the results gathered so far was inconsistent. Many arguments that are close need extensive and costly work that can never be completed. Reasonable guidance would be to eliminate vast quantities of all chemicals that are potentially related to disease, but it could be impossible to do so in diverse, technologically sophisticated industrial communities.

Physical Activity and Cancer Risk

Having mild or intense physical exercise a part of your diet reduces the chances of obesity and other serious illnesses, such as cardiac failure and diabetes. Normal to intense physical activity is a type of workout that helps you sweat and your heart pump quicker. That involves walking, biking, riding, or driving. A increasing body of evidence shows that performing some sort of exercise to prevent too much sitting will help reduce the risk of cancer.

Physical activity can reduce the risk of cancer Evidence suggests that people who exercise regularly are at a lower risk of cancer.

Cancer of the bowel. Research that monitor broad numbers of people over time indicate that persons that workout frequently tend to have a reduced chance of contracting bowel cancer. While we do not say for sure whether exercising itself decreases the incidence of cancer, individuals who exercising frequently have a 40 to 50 per cent greater chance of colon cancer relative to someone who do not exercise regularly. Many research shows that individuals who are involved all their life are at the lowest risk of colon cancer.

Breast cancer: Recent broad, long-term findings indicate that people who participate in mild to intensive activity for more than 3 hours a week have a 30 to 40% reduced chance of breast cancer. It extends to all people, regardless of family background or incidence of breast cancer.

Several findings suggest that the greater the exercise frequency, the lower the chance of cancer. Nevertheless, it is not known if a particular standard of operation has to be achieved to reduce the harm. Exercise is necessary over a person's life, but exercise at any age may help to minimize the risk of breast cancer.

Cancer of the uterine: Some studies have linked exercise to a lower risk of uterine cancer.

Cancer of the heart: Research suggest that daily healthy individuals are less likely to contract lung cancer.

There is a great deal of current work on physical exercise and its impact on disease. Recent work suggests that only moderate exercise can offer certain health benefits. Light movement is something you do to prevent sitting back or laying down.

Children and adolescents In order to promote a lifetime of physical exercise, children and adolescents will remain involved on a daily basis. Physical activity habits that begin in childhood also progress to adulthood. Children will have mild to intense exercise for at least 60 minutes a day. Children and teenagers can be actively involved for at least 3 days a week. Here are some ways in which you can promote behavior in children:

Cut down on TV time

Limit time playing video games

Limit computer use and use of other electronic devices

Participate in sports or fitness activities

Play actively at school or home

CHAPTER TWO
TYPES OF CANCER

There are over 100 forms of cancer. Types of cancer are generally referred to as organs or tissues where cancers are produced. For eg, lung cancer begins in the lung cells, and brain cancer begins in the brain cells. Cancers can often be identified by the type of cells that shaped them, such as epithelial cells or squamous cells.

We do provide a range of details on pediatric tumors and diseases of youth and young adults.

Below are several examples of cancers that begin with different types of cells:

Carcinoma

Carcinoma is the most prevalent form of cancer. These are produced by epithelial cells, which are cells that protect the body's internal and external surfaces. There are many forms of epithelial cells that often have a column-like appearance when presented under a microscope.

Carcinomas that develop in different types of epithelial cells have specific names: adenocarcinoma is a cancer that develops in epithelial cells that produce fluids or mucus. Tissues with this type of epithelial cell are sometimes referred to as glandular tissues. Many breast, bowel, and prostate tumors are adenocarcinomas.

Basal cell carcinoma is a cancer that occurs in the lower or basal (base) layer of the epidermis, which is the outer layer of the skin of a human.

Squamous cell carcinoma is a disease that occurs in squamous cells, epithelial cells that reside just below the exterior surface of the skin. Squamous cells also make out many key tissues, including the heart, intestines, lungs, liver, and kidneys. Squamous cells appear smooth, like a fish scale, when presented under a microscope. Squamous cell carcinomas are often referred to as epidermoid carcinomas.

Transitional cell carcinoma is a cancer that arises in a form of epithelial tissue called a transitional epithelium or urothelium. This tissue, which is made up of several layers of epithelial cells that can develop larger and smaller, is located in the linings of the bladder, ureters, and most of the kidneys (renal pelvis) and a few other organs. Any tumors of the liver, urethra, and kidneys are intermediate cell carcinomas.

Sarcoma

Soft tissue sarcoma develops in the body's soft tissues, including organs, tendons, skin, blood channels, lymphatic channels, nerves, and tissue throughout the joints.

Credit: Teresa Winslow Sarcomas are tumors that arise in bone and soft tissue, including skin, fat, blood channels, lymphatic channels, and fibrous tissue (such as tendons and ligaments).

Osteosarcoma is the most severe bone cancer. Leiomyosarcoma, Kaposi sarcoma, malignant fibrous histiocytoma, liposarcoma, and dermatofibrosarcoma protuberans are the most severe forms of soft tissue sarcoma.

Leukemia

Cancers that begin in the blood-forming tissue of the bone marrow are called leukemia. Such cancers do not form a large tumor. Therefore, vast amounts of rare white blood cells (leukemia cells and leukemia blast cells) make up in the blood and bone marrow, crowding out normal blood cells. Low levels of regular blood cells can make it harder for the body to get oxygen to its tissues, stop bleeding, or combat infections.

There are four popular forms of leukemia which are classified on the basis of how rapidly the condition is becoming worse (acute or chronic) and the type of blood cell in which the cancer occurs (lymphoblastic or myeloid).

Lymphoma

Lymphoma is a cancer that occurs in lymphocytes (T or B cells). That is the disease-fighting of white blood cells that is part of the immune response. In lymphoma, dysfunctional lymphocytes are produced in lymph nodes and lymph tubes, as well as in other organs of the body.

There are two major forms of lymphoma: Hodgkin lymphoma – Patients with this condition have rare lymphocytes called Reed-Sternberg cells. Such cells normally shape B cells.

Non-Hodgkin lymphoma – A broad community of cancers that begin in lymphocytes, Cancers can develop rapidly or gradually and can be produced from B cells or T cells.

Multiple myeloma

Multiple myeloma is a cancer that starts in plasma cells, another form of immune cells. Abnormal plasma cells, or myeloma cells, grow up in the bone marrow and develop bone tumors in the body. Advanced myeloma is often referred to as white cell myeloma and Kahler syndrome.

Melanoma

Melanoma is a disease that starts in cells that are melanocytes, which are advanced cells that produce melanin (a pigment that provides color to the skin). Most melanomas develop on the skin, although melanomas may also grow in other pigmented tissues, such as the hair.

Brain and spinal cord tumors

These are growing forms of brain and spinal cord tumors. Such tumors are identified depending on the type of cell in which they were developed and when the tumor was first developed in the central nervous system. For starters, an astrocytic tumor occurs in star-shaped brain cells called astrocytes that help maintain nerve cells alive. Brain tumors can be benign (not cancer) or malignant (cancer).

Many Tumor Forms Germ Cell

Tumors Germ Cell tumors are a form of tumor that starts in cells that give birth to sperm or eggs. Such tumors may appear nearly everywhere in the body and can be either benign or malignant.

Neuroendocrine

Tumors Neuroendocrine tumors are produced by cells that release hormones into the blood in response to a nervous system signal. These cancers, which can trigger higher-than-normal hormone rates, can trigger several specific symptoms. Neuroendocrine tumors may be benign or malignant.

Carcinoid Tumors

The carcinoid tumor is a form of neuroendocrine tumor. These are slow-growing tumors that are typically located in the gastrointestinal tract (most commonly in the rectum and small intestines). Carcinoid tumors that migrate to the liver or other areas of the body, and may secrete compounds such as serotonin or prostaglandins that induce carcinoid syndrome

Which are the symptoms and indicators of cancer

Symptoms and symptoms of cancer depend on the type of cancer in which it is found and/or where cancer cells have dispersed. Of example, breast cancer can be present as a lump in the breast or as a nipple discharge, whereas metastatic breast cancer can display symptoms of discomfort (if extended to the bones), intense weakness (lungs), or seizures (brain). A few people have no signs or effects until the cancer has spread.

The American Cancer Society identifies seven warning signs and/or symptoms that cancer might be present and this may cause a individual to pursue medical treatment. The term CAUTION will help you understand this things.

- Shift in bowel or bladder patterns

- Sore throat that does not heal

- Irregular bleeding or discharge (for example, nipple secretions or sores that do not cure the material)

- thickening or lumping of the breast, testicles or elsewhere

- Indigestion (usually chronic) or trouble swallowing

- Noticeable improvement in the appearance, colour, form or thickness of the wart or mole

- Nagging cough Which include:

- Unexplained weight loss or lack of appetite

- Different form of bone or certain areas of the body discomfort that can gradually intensify or escalate, which is unlike past symptoms that have existed previously

- Recurrent weakness, diarrhea, or vomiting

- Unexplained low-grade fevers that can be either recurrent or continue on and on

- Recurrent illnesses that do not clear.

Most cancers have any of the above generic signs, but also have one or two signs that are more unique to the form of cancer. For starters, lung cancer may have specific signs of pain, but the pain is generally located in the chest. The patient may experience irregular bleeding, but bleeding typically happens while the patient coughs. Patients with lung cancer frequently become out of breath and often feel really sleepy.

Since there are so many forms of cancer (see next section) and so many non-specific and often more common effects, the easiest approach to know about the signs and symptoms of different types of cancer is to spend a few minutes studying the symptoms of a particular part of the body. Conversely, a different region of the body will be checked to figure out what indications and symptoms a person can watch for in the region suspected of getting cancer.

• Use a search engine (Google, Bing) to locate connections to cancer by describing the signs accompanied by the word "cancer" or if you know the kind of details you seek (lung, head, breast)

For example, the naming of "blood in urine and cancer" would lead a individual to websites that list potential organs and body systems where cancer may trigger the symptoms mentioned.

• Use the search tool as above to mention the identified body region to disease (e.g., bladder and prostate) and the individual can find places that report the indications and symptoms of disease in the region (blood in the urine is one of the few symptoms listed).

• Be mindful that certain databases are not always checked by a health provider and can provide information that is not reliable. In the end, the health care provider is the strongest option if you have questions.

In fact, once the type of cancer is identified (detected), more detailed checks may be made to identify the category of cancer detected and any cancer might be called (symptoms, tumor rates, medications, prognosis, among several other items).

One's own study will not override contact with a health care practitioner if anyone is worried about cancer.

When Cancer Spreads

In metastases, cancer cells split free from where they initially originated (primary cancer), migrate across the blood or lymph system, and develop new tumors (metastatic tumors) in certain areas of the body. The metastatic tumor is the same form of cancer as that of the main tumor.

A cancer that has spread from the location where it began to grow to another position in the body is considered metastatic cancer. The mechanism through which cancer cells migrate to certain areas of the body is called metastases.

Metastatic cancer has the same name and class of cancer cells as the main or primary cancer. For example, breast cancer, which progresses to and develops a metastatic tumor in the abdomen, is metastatic breast cancer, not lung cancer.

Under a microscope, metastatic cancer cells usually behave the same as the original cancer cells. In comparison, metastatic cancer cells and initial cancer cells typically have some molecular features in general, such as the existence of different chromosome shifts.

Treatment can help to extend the lives of some people with

metastatic cancer. By fact, though, the main aim of metastatic cancer therapy is to monitor or reduce the effects of cancer development. Metastatic cancers may do significant harm to the working of the body, and most patients who suffer from cancer suffer from metastatic disease.

CHAPTER THREE
ABOUT HOW TO STARVE CANCER

Cancer cells develop in distinctive ways that contradict typical limitations.

The growth process requires nutrition, and cancer cells metabolize nutrients in specific forms than healthy cells around them. Chemotherapy medications attack certain channels within cancer cells in an effort to destroy the tumor without destroying normally working cells. This is extremely complex, costly and vulnerable to adverse side effects that have triggered most of the disease-related misery.

The value of eating for disorders such as diabetes and hypertension, diagnostics that come with well-known nutritional medications, has long been recognized. Also the most widely prescribed drug in type 2 diabetes, metformin, was shown to be detrimental to diet and exercise in clinical studies. Cell biologists like Locasale see the expansion of this line of thought to cancer as a rational move, since at cellular stage, cancer is actually a metabolic pathway disorder.

Suggesting patients to hurry or starve to kill a tumor has been a controversial and inflated assertion over the years, and this is not the recommendation today. In recent years, metabolic processes have been focused, following diverse approaches to improving what people consume. Several studies included reducing the consumption of sugar. Indeed, certain cancer cells metabolize glucose at higher than average rates (to help the aerobic glycolysis process) and depleting their access to sugar will delay development.

Chemotherapy can be the norm of treatment for certain cases of cancer; however, it may not fully differentiate between healthy or cancerous cells and can kill both. To certain people, such therapies can be crippling and, sadly, provide no promise for a complete recovery from certain forms of cancer.

Starving cancer cells of the tools they need to replicate and grow In order for either healthy cells or cancer cells to replicate, they require DNA building blocks called nucleotides. Cancers need large rates of DNA building blocks to sustain their accelerated development, and by destroying them, cancers that can be prevented from developing in the body.

Dihydroorotate dehydrogenase (DHODH) is an enzyme that is essential to the synthesis of nucleotides. The Bayer-Broad collaboration contributed to an interesting finding that by inhibiting the DHODH enzyme in the body, cancer cells were deprived of adequate quantities of nucleotides and did not begin to develop in the body. This phenomenon is believed to have a far greater impact on cancer cells than on healthy cells, because they have a higher need for DNA building blocks that can not be produced in adequate amounts from the current body supply.

Following this finding, the chemists participating in the Bayer-Broad partnership set out to find a powerful and unique inhibitor of DHODH that would make it safe for human use. A collaborative initiative also contributed to the discovery of a therapeutic nominee.

Acute myeloid leukemia (AML) is one form of cancer of shared concern in the Bayer-Broad relationship. During this disease, the cells of the bone marrow, or myeloid cells, are malignant and develop tumors. The prevailing quality of treatment is radiation, which puts tremendous pressure on the patient.

The DHODH inhibitor candidate is currently in phase I clinical research, where protection and early indicators of effectiveness are tested in patients with cancers such as AML. We aim to have a new treatment alternative for a wide variety of AML patients. In relation to AML, we are looking at the ability of the drug candidate to suppress the development of solid tumors such as colorectal cancer and non-Hodgkin lymphoma.

There's a scientific experiment going on among us that can show you how to kill cancer cells spontaneously by manipulating something called angiogenesis.

Angiogenesis is a common mechanism utilized by our bodies to create blood vessels.

There are more than 60,000 miles worth of blood arteries in the human body. To help you imagine what an amazing figure that is, remember that 60,000 miles worth of something is enough miles to orbit the planet twice.

Angiogenesis helps the body to build blood vessels that can be tailored to some form of disease in the human body. When this is not controlled, it can induce overgrowth of diseases such as obesity, blindness, endometriosis of arthritis, and multiple sclerosis. It is because the angiogenesis system can produce defects which, in effect, can trigger long-term health problems.

In order to avoid and regulate angiogenesis, it is necessary to understand how to stave cancer cells naturally. According to revered Dr. Li, "Angiogenesis is the primary cause of all cancers." Cancer cells can not develop into big, life-threatening tumors without adequate numbers of capillaries that provide a lot of oxygen and nutrient-rich blood.

There are over 19 billion capillaries, the smallest blood arteries of the entire body. If such capillaries grow out of balance owing to a faulty angiogenesis mechanism, cancer is likely to occur.

Most people travel about every day bearing unseen, undeveloped microscopic cancer cell clusters. Fortunately for human beings, as long as the body retains the potential to adequately regulate angiogenesis, it can keep the blood vessels from expanding to fuel such small tumors.

Anti-angiogenic treatment is a tool to reduce the blood flow of small colonies of cancer cells over time. It is likely since the tumor structures are extremely irregular and badly designed, rendering them very susceptible to care approaches that specifically kill them.

There are hundreds of various anti-angiogenic cancer medications that, according to Doctor Li, have dramatically improved survival levels in cancer patients, but perhaps more relevant are the methods to starve cancer spontaneously before it grows. "The key approach used to starve angiogenesis is to ingest a vast number of super-foods that have the ability to starve microscopic cancerous development. There are several plants, beverages, and diets that are naturally available and have the strength and capacity to prevent angiogenesis.

Eating these super foods will strengthen the body's self-regulation mechanism and keep blood vessels from growing and feeding small tumors that occur in most humans at any given time.

When the connection between obesity and metabolic syndrome and cancer is clearer, it is becoming more necessary to determine the best approach to implement dietary therapy in the care of cancer patients. Metabolic-based treatments, such as dietary restriction, prolonged fasting and ketogenic diet, have the potential to decrease the occurrence of random tumors and delay the development of primary tumors, which could have an impact on distant metastases in animal models. Given the plethora of preclinical evidence showing the value of cancer dietary change, there are currently few clinical studies investigating food as an intervention in cancer patients. We hypothesize that this could be attributed, in part, to the fact that there are many specific methods of dietary change without any consistent guidelines on the best process.

What kind of diet is anti-angiogneic?

A strong example of anti-angiogenic products can be contained in red grapes.

Red grapes produce resveratrol, a fat-soluble compound present in the flesh.

According to Dr. Li, Reveratrol has been shown to suppress pathological angiogenesis by 60 percent. In recent years, a growing number of experiments have demonstrated that resveratrol induces a particular form of death in cancer-containing cells.

The greatest aspect of the anti-angiogenic diet is that it appears to be tasty. Cherries, strawberries, blackberries, raspberries and blueberries are full of anti-angiogenic energy. Comfortable foods, such as green tea and red wine, often have anti-angiogenic effects. Cooking ingredients such as tomatoes, artichokes, kale, garlic, parsley, turmeric and maitake mushrooms are not only simple to include in nearly any meal, but they do possess potent anti-angiogenic properties.

The true force behind starving cancer spontaneously through anti-angiogenic drugs is not to choose one diet or drink to improve the body's innate capacity to control the angiogenic response, but the incredible teamwork that occurs when you do it together. As a consequence, not only do you stop packaged products, you build a whole diet full of healthy ingredients.

You might be curious whether this therapy will be as successful as using potent poisonous medications that are both anti-angiogenic. Okay, according to Dr. Li, there are several foods that have been proven to be just as safe. Foods such as red grapes, parsley and garlic have similar anti-angiogenic potency relative to other anti-angiogenic products, albeit without adverse consequences.

How cancer cells fuel their growth

Cancer cells are infamous for being able to fragment uncontrollably and produce hordes of fresh tumor cells. Some of the food that these quickly proliferating cells eat is glucose, a form of sugar.

Scientists claimed that much of the mass of cells that made up individual cells, including cancer cells, originated from glucose. Nevertheless, to their disappointment, MIT scientists have now discovered that the main type of new cell content is amino acids, which cells absorb in far smaller amounts.

The results provide a fresh way of looking at the metabolism of cancer cells, a area of science that scientists hope will create innovative medicines that can cut off the capacity of cancer cells to expand and split.

"When you want to effectively approach cancer metabolism, you need to consider how various mechanisms are primarily used to produce mass.

Burning up

Since the 1920s, scientists have understood that cancer cells produce energy differently from regular cells, a process named the "Warburg Influence" after its discoverer, the German biochemist Otto Warburg. Human cells usually utilize glucose as an energy source, which is broken down by a sequence of complicated chemical reactions involving oxygen. Warburg discovered that tumor cells are transitioning to a less effective biochemical technique known as fermentation, which does not need oxygen and consumes even less electricity.

More recently, scientists have proposed that cancer cells utilize this alternate mechanism to establish building blocks for new cells. One criticism against this theory, though, is that a significant portion of glucose is transformed into lactate, a waste substance that is not suitable for cells. In fact, relatively little work has been performed about just what is involved in the formation of modern cancer cells or some type of quickly dividing mammalian cells.

"Since animals consume such a large variety of foods, it seems like an open problem as to which diet relates to certain sections of the mass.

Scientists have developed many various kinds of cancer cells and regular cells in culture dishes to establish which cells, including those in tumors, were receiving the building blocks they required. We fed various nutrients labelled with alternative sources of carbon and nitrogen to the cells, enabling them to watch where the initial molecules ended up. They also measured the cells before and after they were separated, enabling them to measure the amount of cell mass added by each of the usable nutrients.

While the cells absorb glucose and amino acid glutamine at very large levels, the researchers noticed that these two molecules contribute little to the mass of fresh cells — Glucose accounts for 10 to 15 per cent of the carbon noticed in the cells, whereas glutamine contributes only 10 per cent of the carbon. Instead, the main contributors of cell mass were the amino acids that made up proteins. As a category, amino acids (excluding glutamine) add much of the carbon atoms present in fresh cells and 20 to 40 per cent of the overall mass. While initially shocking, the results make sense, Vander Heiden says, since cells are mainly composed of protein.

"There's a sort of system utilizing a cheaper, more straightforward path to create what you're made of," he says. "If you choose to create a house out of bricks, it's better if you have a ton of bricks surrounding you to using certain bricks than beginning with dirt to creating fresh bricks." Refocusing the problem It's always a mystery why proliferating human cells eat too much glucose. Consistent with previous findings, researchers have observed that most glucose consumed by these cells is excreted as lactate.

"This has led us to believe that the value of high glucose intake is not simply the exploitation of carbon that enables cell mass to be generated, but rather for other items that it supplies, such as electricity,

Steps for starving cancer

Another successful strategy to combat cancer for people with defective genetics or immune systems is to kill cancer cells, stopping them from spreading. For eg, reducing or removing sugar, including sugar substitutes, as well as replacing traditional salt with sea salt. Ingestion of milk creates mucosa in the gastrointestinal tract, thus removing milk and replacing it with soya, which may tend to starve cancer cells. Most notably, red meat foods are rich in acidity and cancer cells flourish in acidic conditions. Food frequently includes hormones, toxins and viruses that are very dangerous to the flesh. However, unlike food, high protein in meat is difficult to digest and needs multiple digestive enzymes.

Food that is not digested persists in the stomach and rots that transform into other poisonous materials. Talk of consuming fish or poultry instead of beef. Ideally, a diet full of fruits, grains, foods, nuts and berries is strongly recommended. New vegetable juices have strong enzymes that are quickly absorbed to the cellular level in 15 minutes, nourishing and promoting the development of healthy cells.

At the main, cancer is a disorder of mind, body, and soul. Positive action allows a individual with cancer to live as rage and pessimistic thoughts place the body in an acidic climate. Because cancer cells do not survive in an oxygenated environment, regular activity and controlled breathing are strongly recommended. Even, stop placing food in disposable pots or disposable wrappings in a microwave oven. Under extreme pressure, plastic produces dioxins, a cancerous compound that penetrates the food you're cooking up.

Further recommendations are:

[1] Consume a range of fresh products that contain strong and healthy antioxidants that are outstanding in detoxifying our body system from chronic toxemia and acidosis. Drink enough healthy, unpolluted air to help filter away waste materials.

[2] It is recommended to consume more locally produced vegetables and fruit, 5 servings of vegetables and 3 servings of fruit each day. Only eaten untreated, high in life-enhancing enzymes. Be sure they're grown organically.

[3] Ingest more beans or legumes that will help avoid mutations in cells[4] Be mindful of our weight, don't overeat or stuff yourself, most instances of cancer are attributed to overeating with incorrect foods and beverages. [Mandarin term cancer consists of three mouths that make up the peak, implying overeating][5] Exercise mildly, go for relaxing and good breathing, and make sure that our body cells are well irrigated with oxygen and dispose of waste items.

[6] Should not consume burned food or old fat. Fats quickly go wrong and become toxic and produce carcinogens when overheated or disrupted. [Beware of groundnuts, abundant in fats, but when such fats become skewed or old, they taste bad, they don't consume] [7] Consume meats or seafood sparingly [too acidic in nature] [8] Keep from consuming too much alcohol, stop smoking [don't kill our body intentionally] [9] Don't eat dried, refined, frozen products heavy in carcinogens or preservatives, chemical flavourings and coloring.

There are other explanations that are not used or clarified. Yet you may have read about it. 'Starve cancer cells,' should not feed them with animal proteins. Get to learn the wonder sprouts that produce strong phyto-factors that will improve one's immune system. Prevention is far easier than treatment. Spend our capital carefully, do not purchase 'troubles,' do not 'invite' it.

Humans don't get ill naturally, generally. Humans are incredibly resilient and solid and stable, so we do not deliberately infect ourselves with unsuitable food that induces toxemia and acidosis. Be grateful that our heart has been pumping blood through our circulatory system since we were raised. Be grateful that our hearts, our kidneys, and our livers all worked for us for many years. Our kidneys will still function even though they are left with a 5 percent power.

They will take proactive steps. It's never too complicated or too far out or unlikely! Don't feel so naive that the 'ghost of suffering' isn't going to hit someone. Don't plan a situation that invites us. Don't welcome, just scare it out, store it with a good immune system, and again be grateful that we have lots of food, fruits and herbs that will eliminate cancer at first. Indeed, there are cancer-preventing products very close to us.

If there are foods that can cause cancer, there are also other foods that can prevent cancer, be mindful of this reality.

Starving Of Cancer With Power Foods

There are certain products classified as "strength food" that have a good resistance against cancer. Such strength products are classified as 'phytonutrients.

(1) Isoflavones :- isoflavones are active estrogens present in soybean and soy products. It has cancer-fighting powers. Some research in China have shown that routine intake of soybean products decreases the incidence of stomach, breast, uterus, colon and lung cancer. At least two anticacinogens have been found in soybean. That contains isoflavones and saponins. Therefore, in an effort to combat and avoid cancer, the soya bean food will be a daily diet. Those include

   I.   Roasted soy nuts

   II.   Soya bean flour

   III. Soya bean cheese

(iv) Soya bean milk at least one cup a day. Anything you can do with soybean, it's good. Only keep consuming all sorts of soya bean items. Why is the soy drug working? You ought to realize that cancer develops fresh blood vessels so that they can begin to expand and feed their control cells. Soya bean is a potent phytonutrient that also prevents the development of these fresh blood vessels and thus starves the tumors. Soya phytoestrogen directly blocks the capacity of cancer cells to replicate and develop into tumors.

(2) Some of the other phytonutrients are a. Lycopene, which can be derived from untreated TOMATOES. This is an antioxidant that helps avoid cancer and protect the skin.

a. Sulphoraphane :- available in broccoli that helps avoid cancer and detoxify cells. Polyphebnol :- These are usable GREEN TEA, and also helps resist antibacterial detoxification by cancer. Organo-sulfur :- These are used in GARLIC to improve the immune system e. Flavonoids; found in raw Onions and Apples for the protection of the heart and prevention of cancer.

f. Ellagic-Acid :- Available in bananas, grapes and walnuts, both of which possess anti-cancer properties.

Many tips to starve cancer

1. Stop saturated fat that comes from food foods such as raw milk, bacon, red meat, poultry, chocolate, ice cream, butter, margarine.

2. Stop the fat that is unhealthy. Be mindful of the amount and quantity of oil you drink 3. Omega 3 fatty acids are a healthy replacement that will benefit. This is also found in raw nuts such as walnut, linseed, and found in certain fresh mackerel. It is found in most aquatic plants.

3. Extra virgin olive oil is the perfect spot to prepare

4. Consume a lot of food that is a full plant based diet,

vegetable & fruit such as mango, banana, maize, beans, peppers, almonds, carrots, green beans, peaches, onions, strawberries, cabbage, spinach, tomatoes, watermelons, pink grapefruit, squash, etc.

5. Drink half a cup of new carrot juice per day. It's a good antioxidant that protects against cancer. You need a juicer to get the carrot juice out of the plant, cabbage juice even prevents cancer.

6. Detoxify the liver with a cup of hot water mixed with sugar, first thing in the morning. It's an ideal stimulant to flush the liver.

7. Take at least 3 liters of water a day, stop chlorine-containing liquids. Chlorine is a material that induces cancer.

8. Choose herbal tea with new mint leaves instead of coffee 10. Eliminate sugar sweetened foods from your diet 11. Raw fresh tomatoes produce glycogen, a big antioxidant that prevents prostate cancer, so consume a lot of raw fresh tomatoes 12. Take certain vitamins such as Glutamine, 30 minutes before your meal, Vitamin A, Beta Carotene, Vitamin C, Folic Acid, Calcium etc. Contact the doctor before taking any medication.

9. Apply Scottish sea salt to the food, not sodium chloride or table salt.

10. Remove all dried, jarred, packaged, and even frozen items that are very harmful.

11. Making sure you're getting a lot of new garlic. Drink a

ton of new garlic & ginger drink Note: do not chew or swallow garlic. It should be ground and dissolved in water for optimum gain. There is nothing we eat that is more detrimental to our wellbeing than livestock products, none at all!

Tissue modifications that are not cancer

Not every shift in body tissue is cancer. However, certain tissue changes can turn into cancer if they are not treated. Here are some instances of tissue alterations that are not disease but are in some situations monitored: hyperplasia happens as cells in the tissue grow more than average and excess cells build up or proliferate. But, under a microscope, the cells and the way the tissue is arranged appear natural. Hyperplasia can be induced by a variety of causes or disorders, including persistent discomfort.

Dysplasia is more severe than hyperplasia. There is also an aggregation of excess cells in dysplasia. But the cells appear irregular and there are shifts in the way the tissue is arranged. In fact, the more unhealthy the cells and tissues appear, the greater the risk that cancer may arise.

Some forms of dysplasia can need to be controlled or treated. An indication of dysplasia is an irregular mole (called a dysplastic nevus) developed on the skin. A dysplastic nevus can develop into melanoma, although most may not.

Carcinoma in situ is an even more serious condition. Although it is often referred to as cancer, carcinoma in situ is not cancer since abnormal cells do not grow beyond the initial tissue. This is, they don't enter surrounding tissues the way cancer cells do. Nevertheless, since certain in situ carcinomas may become cancer, they are typically treated.

Normal cells can become cancer cells. Until cancer cells develop in the body's tissues, the cells experience pathological modifications termed hyperplasia and dysplasia. During hyperplasia, there is an spike in the amount of cells in the organ or tissue that tend to be normal under a microscope. For dysplasia, the cells appear strange under the microscope, but they are not cancerous. Hyperplasia and dysplasia may or may not turn into cancer.

Cancer cells thriving on a mistake

Approximately 85-90 per cent of cancer cells contain the incorrect amount of chromosomes. Yet how are they to live and evolve under these conditions?

Anomaly as a particular function The starting point for a study that explores the basic processes of cell division. ecause chromosomes include genes, the architecture of humans, "each of the daughter cells of the dividing cell requires the right and equivalent complement of chromosomes, n onetheless, often the daughter cells wind up having the incorrect amount of chromosomes.

Generally, this so-called aneuploid condition is dangerous, sometimes lethal to the embryo – it may contribute to pregnancy or developmental defects such as Down's Syndrome in very early life. Nevertheless, this does not appear to extend to cancer cells that live and often grow in these circumstances.

The origins of chromosome division errors and their effect on the daughter cells are still unknown. As long as cancer cells are concerned, we will not know if this is something advantageous to cancer, or if it is either another form of mutation identical to other cancer-causing mutations, or if it is a recurrence to certain stages to cancer growth, and therefore something the cells need to solve." In the years to come, the work would investigate the fundamental processes of chromosome division and differentiation. It, he believes, would offer a deeper glimpse into the nature of cancer as well as other fields of study. "Chromosomes are a very important feature of all cells.

A deeper knowledge of how they function will have an effect on almost every area in biology." For example, the process in cell division right before chromosomes break apart would be of special importance. Typically, there are processes that "distinguish between chromosomes that are correctly balanced and those that are misaligned and thus need to be fixed." Nevertheless, such processes often do not operate.

A protein named P53 is essential for the production of aneuploid cells. Although it normally suggests errors in the DNA of a cell, the overwhelming majority of cancer cells have interrupted its function. "But that's obviously not the whole story. Because you get a third copy of a chromosome, all the genes on it are expressed about 50% more. There are thousands of genes on a chromosome, each having a little bit of a contribution to the destruction of cell activity." Compared to bacteria, the mechanism of chromosome division in yeast cells is more intricate but not too difficult for an outsider. In comparison, in relation to much more sophisticated mammalian cells, nascent yeast helps researchers to easily produce outcomes. "In a month, the cells have been through hundreds of years. We will see at a very basic level how they have developed to possessing the incorrect number of chromosomes.

CHAPTER FOUR
UNDERSTANDING CANCER RISK

Risk is a possibility that an incident is going to happen. While thinking about disease, the possibility is often commonly used to define a person's likelihood of having disease. This is often used to identify the risk of the cancer returning or repeating.

Scientists and clinicians utilize cancer incidence to enhance the health of other individuals. Another example of that is knowing the dangers of smoke. Researchers have noticed that smoking raises the incidence of lung cancer. We also used this awareness to initiate a national anti-smoking initiative to help save lives.

Knowing risk factors A risk factor for cancer is something that raises a person's likelihood of developing cancer. Nonetheless, most risk factors do not specifically affect cancer. Many patients with a variety of risk factors never grow cancer. And those with no established risk factors do this.

It's important to learn the risk factors and speak to your health care team about them. It will help you make healthier decisions regarding your lifestyle and enhance your safety. Such knowledge can even help the doctor determine whether you require genetic tests and recommendations.

Common warning factors for cancer include: older age Recent or social history of cancer Usage of cigarettes Smoking Drugs Many forms of viral diseases, such as human papillomavirus (HPV) Certain substances Uv damage, including ultraviolet radiation, can be prevented by avoiding unhealthy behaviors.

Those involve the use of cigarettes and alcohol, overweight, and frequent sunburns. Certain contributing factors, such as becoming older, can not be minimized. Know more regarding the risk factors for other forms of cancer.

Likelihood factors and cancer screening Knowing the risk of cancer will help the doctor determine if you could gain from: a cancer screening examination, such as mammogram or colonoscopy A screening procedure at an early age and more frequently than regular screening Treatment or medications to minimize the risk of cancer For example, a woman whose mother has breast cancer is at least twice as likely to develop cancer. Many may have a clear family background or hereditary disorder correlated with breast cancer. Because they are at a very high risk of breast cancer, they can opt to shave their breasts in order to avoid cancer. This surgery tends to raise the chance of breast cancer by at least 95%. Some people can often opt to take medicine to reduce the risk of breast cancer.

Individuals with a long family history of cancer will suggest genetic testing. The psychiatrist or genetic advisor will speak to you for any genetic tests. We will inform you the likelihood of getting cancer depending on your family background and other risk factors.

Understanding the distinction between extreme and relative risks Extreme risks and relative risks are used by doctors to determine whether a person's risk is greater or lower than that of either the general public or a particular category of individuals.

Absolute risk is a probability that a individual may contract a disease in a specified period. It determines how many individuals are at risk of contracting a illness in the general community.

Consider, for example, the assertion "1 out of 8 women (12.5%) may develop breast cancer in their lifetime," which defines the actual danger to the general population of women. It can not define the danger to a single individual or community of people. Of example, an actual probability can not be seen that a group of older people has a greater chance of breast cancer than a group of younger people.

Relative risk measures the probability of sickness between two sets of individuals. This contrasts the probability of one group with a certain risk factor for a disease to another group.

Suppose, for example, if you equate the likelihood of breast cancer for two classes of 100 people. Nevertheless, only people in 1 category have a certain risk factor for breast cancer. The other category of people may not have this risk factor. Scientists maintain track of how many individuals in each population grow cancer over a span of time. Let's assume the two people who have the same risk factor have cancer. Yet only one woman lacking this risk factor has cancer. Then people in the first category have 2 times the chance of the second tier. It is a 100% rise in perceived danger. The actual chance, though, will be 2% or 2 out of 100 men.

Patients can use risk assessments to make smarter decisions regarding lifestyle improvements or cancer screening. This is therefore necessary to recognize the distinction between actual and conditional threats. For eg, the relative risk in the last eg may sound big. The relative probability of a individual contracting cancer was defined by 100 per cent. But look at the utter cost of a more full image. That's 1 human in 100, compared to 2 in 100. When you choose to equate the work you've read about in the press with your own case, make sure you consider the maximum chance. The bulk of academic studies assess relative risks. This can make the probability sound greater than it really is.

Cancer statistics

Cancer has a significant influence on people in the United States and around the globe. Cancer reports explain what occurs in broad numbers of individuals and offer a realistic description of the effect of cancer on society. Statistics inform us details about how many patients are born and died with cancer per year, the number of people still surviving under cancer treatment, the total age of treatment, and the percentage of people already alive at the point of diagnosis. We also warn us about disparities between age groups, genders, racial / ethnic classes, regional areas, and other categories.

While clinical patterns are typically not specifically relevant to particular people, it is important for policymakers, decision leaders, health practitioners and academics to consider the effect of cancer on the community and to establish approaches to tackle the threats that cancer presents to society at large. Statistical patterns are often critical for evaluating the progress of cancer prevention and management efforts.

Statistics at a glance: Risk of Cancer in the United States

- An unprecedented 1,735,350 new cases of cancer will be reported in the United States in 2018 and 609,640 individuals will suffer from the disease.

- Breast cancer, lung and bronchus cancer, prostate cancer, colon and rectal cancer, skin melanoma, cervical cancer, non-Hodgkin lymphoma, renal and pelvic cancer, endometrial cancer, leukemia, pancreatic cancer, thyroid cancer, and liver cancer are the most widespread cancers (listed in decreasing order according to estimated new cases in 2018).

- The rate of reported cases of cancer (cancer incidence) is 439.2 per 100,000 males and females each year (based on 2011–2015 reports).

- The rate of cancer deaths (cancer mortality) is 163.5 per 100,000 males and females per year (based on 2011–2015 deaths).

- Cancer incidence in men is greater than among women (196.8 per 100,000 males and 139.6 per 100,000 females). By contrasting race / ethnicity and sex classes, cancer incidence is greatest among African American males (239.9 per 100,000) and lowest for Asian / Pacific Islander people (88.3 per 100,000).

- An additional 15.5 million cancer patients were found in the United States in 2016. The number of cancer patients is projected to climb to 20.3 million by 2026.

- Nearly 38.4 per cent of men and women would be infected with cancer at any stage in their lifespan (based on statistics from 2013–2015).

- A record 15,270 children and teenagers aged 0 to 19 were diagnosed with cancer in 2017 and 1,790 died of the disease.

- Total gross spending on cancer treatment in the United States in 2017 was $147.3 billion. Costs are expected to rise in coming years as society ages and the incidence of cancer rises. Costs are also expected to escalate when modern and much more costly procedures are embraced when quality of care.

- Statistics at a glance: Risk of Cancer Worldwide

- Cancer is one of the leading causes of death worldwide. There were 14.1 million reported diagnoses and 8.2 million cancer-related deaths globally in 2012.

- 57% of new cancer diagnoses emerged in 2012 in less established areas of the world, including Central America and portions of Africa and Asia; 65 percent of cancer deaths have emerged in these areas.

- The rate of reported cases of cancer is projected to increase to 23.6 million a year by 2030.

U.S.— Cancer mortality Trends A decrease in age-adjusted mortality (death) levels is the main predictor of success toward cancer, while other metrics, such as quality of life, are still significant. Incidence is always significant, but it is not always simple to understand shifts in incidence. Of example, because a modern diagnostic procedure predicts several instances of cancer that should otherwise have created a issue in someone's life (called overdiagnosis), the prevalence of the cancer will tend to escalate even though the mortality rate would not alter. Nevertheless, a rise in prevalence may also represent a real increase in illness, as is the case when increased exposure to a risk factor triggers more cases of cancer. In this case, the increased incidence is expected to lead to an increase in cancer mortality.

The average mortality rate of cancer in the United States has declined since the early 1990s. The most recent SEER Cancer Statistics Review, published in April 2018, shows that cancer death rates have decreased by: • 1.8 per cent per year for men from 2006 to 2015 • 1.4 per cent per year for women from 2006 to 2015 • 1.4 per cent per year for children aged 0 to 19 from 2011 to 2015 Although death rates for many different types of cancer have also decreased, rates for a few stabi cancers have decreased.

As the average mortality rate of cancer has declined, the percentage of cancer survivors has increasing. Recent findings indicate that progress is being made toward the epidemic, but a lot of research needs to be completed. While smoking rates, a major cause of cancer, have declined, the U.S. population is aging and cancer rates are rising with age. Obesity, another contributing factor for obesity, is also on the rise.

Surveillance, Epidemiology, and End Results (SEER) Program NCI Surveillance, Epidemiology, and End Results (SEER) Program gathers and reports cancer incidence and survival results from community-based cancer registries that represent about 28 per cent of the U.S. population. The SEER software website provides more comprehensive cancer data, including demographic figures for specific forms of cancer, personalized graphs and charts, and interactive resources.

The Regional Cancer Status Assessment Study offers an ongoing summary on the prevalence, survival and patterns of cancer in the United States. This report is jointly authored by experts from NCI, the Centers for Disease Control and Prevention, American Cancer Society, and the North American Association of Central Cancer Registries.

Cancer Disparities

Cancer impacts many ethnic classes in the United States of America. However, certain individuals can have a higher risk of cancer relative to other individuals.

Cancer inequalities (sometimes referred to as cancer risk discrepancies) are variations in cancer indicators such as:

- Frequency (new cases)

- Occurrence (all current cases)

- Mortality (deaths)

- Morbidity (cancer-related health complications)

- Recovery or quality of life following cancer care

- burden of cancer or associated health problems

- test levels

- Cancer-based detection step

While differences are sometimes seen in the sense of race / ethnicity, certain demographic groups can encounter cancer disparities. Those involve categories identified by illness, gender / sexual orientation, geographical place, employment, schooling and other characteristics.

Contributing Factors Inequalities in cancer are believed to represent the interplay of socio-economic influences, community, lifestyle, tension, the climate and biology.

Racial / ethnic minority communities in the United States are more likely to be disadvantaged and under-served (i.e. to have less to no exposure to adequate health services) than whites, so insufficient access to affordable health insurance is a significant contributor to inequalities. For example, because of their racial / ethnic context, the vulnerable and the medically underserved are less likely to get cancer screening testing than those who are medically well supported. They are therefore more likely to be infected with late-stage cancer that may have been treated more successfully if detected sooner.

Higher cancer risks in disadvantaged and underserved populations can also represent specific levels of cancer risk behavioral influences, such as higher smoking rates, physical inactivity, obesity, and unnecessary alcohol consumption, and lower breast-feeding rates. In comparison, individuals residing in poverty that face higher levels of exposure to environmental risk factors, such as cancer-causing pollutants in motor vehicle emissions in dense urban areas.

Many racial / ethnic minority groups can suffer cancer inequalities even among people of higher socio-economic status. Such discrepancies that indicate cultural disparities such as distrust of the health care system, fatalistic attitudes towards disease, or anxiety or shame towards some forms of medical procedures, these can also indicate regional or other disparities in access to quality treatment.

Disparities in cancer can also indicate disparities in involvement in the clinical study. Clinical studies also have poor attendance among racial / ethnic minorities, which gives rise to the likelihood that the findings will not be entirely relevant to them.

Biological variations often tend to have a part to play in some of the cancer inequalities. Advances in genomics and other genetic innovations are enhancing our knowledge of how biological variations within demographic groups lead to health inequality and how biological influences communicate with other theoretically important variables, such as nutrition and the environment.

For example, some research indicates that there are hereditary or other biological variations between triple-negative breast, colorectal, and prostate cancers that occur in African Americans and those that occur in people of other racial / ethnic groups, and that such variations that explain disparities in the occurrence or aggressiveness of such cancers.

Types of Disparities in Cancer cases

Cancer mortality inequalities arise because there are higher rates of new diagnosis and death levels of cancer within some races, ethnicities, or other demographic groups. Post this video to help people think about cancer treatment disparities in the

United States.

While the prevalence of cancer and total mortality are decreasing among all racial / ethnic categories in the United States, certain populations tend to be at an higher risk of contracting or dying from particular cancers.

Many of the primary cancer prevalence and mortality differences amongst U.S. racial / ethnic populations include:

- African Americans have greater death levels than all other races with many, though not all, types of cancer.

- African American women are also more likely than white people to suffer from breast cancer. The mortality disparity is increasing as the death rate in African-American women, which in the past was lower than in white people, has increased to that of white women.

- African Americans are more than half as likely to die of breast cancer than whites and about twice as likely to die of stomach cancer.

- The prevalence of colorectal cancer is greater in African Americans than in whites. The prevalence of both classes is decreasing, but there is always a disparity between the categories.

- Hispanic and American Indian / Alaska Native women have greater prevalence of cervical cancer than other racial / ethnic groups; African American people have the lowest rates of death from the condition.

American Indians / Alaska Natives report the largest levels of liver and intrahepatic bile duct cancer, led by Asian / Pacific Islanders and Hispanics.

- American Indians / Alaska Natives have higher levels of mortality from kidney cancer than most racial / ethnic categories.

- Both the prevalence of lung cancer and the mortality rate of the disease was greater in African American men than in members of other racial / ethnic groups.

- Some prominent indicators of inequalities include:

- The prevalence levels of colorectal, lung and cervical cancer are far greater in the Rural parts of Ohio than in the poorer and more populous regions of the state.

- African American women are about twice as likely to be infected with triple-negative breast cancer as white women, and is more serious and more challenging to cure than other subtypes of breast cancer.

- African Americans are more than twice as likely to be afflicted with multiple myeloma than whites. Blacks in the United States and Africa still have a greater prevalence of disease labeled monoclonal gammopathy of undetermined meaning (MGUS) than whites, and may be a trigger of multiple myeloma. The disparity is more prominent in younger people.

- There are significant gaps between racial / ethnic classes in the prevalence of colorectal cancer screening, with Spanish-speaking Hispanics less likely to be screened than white or English-speaking Hispanics.

- The incidence of colorectal cancer deaths for those younger than 65 ('premature' deaths) are higher in countries with the lowest level of education than in those with higher levels of education. People with more qualifications are less likely to die early from colorectal cancer than people with fewer experience, irrespective of race or ethnicity.

- Activities that raise the likelihood of cancer, such as smoking and consuming alcohol, could be more common among lesbian, homosexual, and bisexual youth than among heterosexual youth.

Addressing Cancer Disparities

Since several various causes can exacerbate cancer disparities — in particular, deprivation and the associated lack of adequate medical care — it is not easy or clear to fix them. Nonetheless, scholars are finding strategies to tackle the most important causes in social inequalities and are also seeing some impact.

One solution is to tackle access to treatment in particular. For example, in 2002, Delaware set up a state-wide colorectal cancer screening initiative to resolve the inequalities in colorectal cancer among African Americans, which provided for screening and treatment, and rendered patient navigators accessible to organize screening and cancer care. By 2009, this initiative had reversed the disparities in test rates, lowered the number of African Americans infected with cancer that had already advanced, and almost entirely erased racial / ethnic inequalities in prevalence and mortality of colorectal cancer. Numerous initiatives are ongoing to tackle the spread of cancer in rural communities.

Researchers are now discussing biological variations in cancer through racial / ethnic categories. For example, genetic variations are known that could explain the higher incidence of prostate cancer among African American males relative to white males. Researchers are now looking into certain genetic variations that could justify why African American males appear to have more severe prostate cancers than white males. Research of this kind can ultimately help to find approaches to minimize risk in African American people.

How health services find cancer

Any tumors are detected through regular screening tests. These are typically measures that are regularly conducted at a certain level. Many tumors are found as you show clear signs to a health care provider.

Physical examination and medical background, particularly the background of symptoms, are the first steps to diagnosis cancer. For certain cases, a variety of scans may be required by the professional caregiver, several of which will be decided by the form of cancer and where it is believed to be found in or on the body of the individual. In addition, most carers may prescribe a full blood count, electrolyte rates and, in certain instances, other blood tests that can include supplementary detail.

Imaging tests are widely used to help doctors identify anomalies that could be disease in the body. X-ray, CT and MRI scans and ultrasound are standard devices used to analyze the body. Some examinations, such as endoscopy, which can enable the analysis of tissues in the intestinal tract, chest, and bronchial tract that might be cancerous with differences of the equipment used. Radionuclide screening is also used in locations that can not be easily visualized (within bones or certain lymph nodes, for example). The procedure requires the absorption or IV infusion of a weakly toxic material that can be absorbed and observed in irregular tissues.

Past studies can be very effective at localizing irregularities in the body; other doctors find that some of the measures offer conclusive proof for the diagnosis of cancer. Nevertheless, in almost all cases, the final diagnosis of cancer is focused on the analysis of a tissue sample obtained in a test called a tissue biopsy that could be cancerous and subsequently examined by a pathologist. Many biopsy samples are fairly easy to collect (e.g., skin biopsy or intestinal tissue biopsy using an endoscope called a biopsy device). Certain biopsies can involve as little as a closely controlled knife, or as much as surgery (e.g. brain tissue or lymph node biopsy). For certain situations, surgery to diagnose cancer can result in a cure if all cancer tissue is extracted at the time of the biopsy.

Biopsy may include more than a conclusive diagnosis of cancer; it may classify the form of cancer (for example, the form of tissue detected that suggest that the sample is from the main [started there] or metastatic phase of brain cancer [disseminated from another main tumor in another section of the body]) and thereby help to stage cancer. The level, or level of cancer, is a means for doctors and physicians to measure the degree of cancer in the patient's body.

Is the cancer that has been detected localized to its origin location, or is it distributed from that location to other tissues? Localized cancer is considered to be at an early level, whereas one that has progressed is at an advanced point.

How doctors assess the level of cancer

There are a variety of common treatment strategies used by tumors, and the basic treatment requirements varies between forms of cancer. According to the NCI, the specific features found in most staging schemes are as follows:

- Primary tumor location

- Tumor scale and amount of tumors

- Lymph node presence (spreading of cancer into lymph nodes)

- Cell form and tumor classification (how much cancer cells mimic regular tissue cells)

- Identification or lack of metastases

Furthermore, there are two primary factors that make up the tumor. TMN classification is used by most solid tumors, whereas the Roman numeral or stage grouping form is utilized by certain physicians and researchers by nearly all forms of cancer.

The TNM method is focused on the size of the tumor (T), the

magnitude of the spread to the lymph nodes (N) and the existence of remote metastases (M). A number is attached to each letter to signify the size or magnitude of the main tumor and the degree of the spread of cancer (higher number indicates larger tumor or further spread).

The following is the NCI's explanation of the TNM staging system:

1. Primary tumor (T) or TX-Primary tumor can not be examined o T0-No proof of primary tumor o Tis-Carcinoma in situ (CIS); irregular cells are present but have not spread to neighboring tissues; while not cancer, CIS growing become cancer and is often referred to as pre-invasive cancer) o T1, T2, T3, T4-Size and/or magnitude of primary tumor

2. Regional lymph nodes (N) or NX-Regional lymph nodes can not be determined o N0-No regional lymph node presence o N1, N2, N3-Involvement of regional lymph nodes (number of lymph nodes and/or degree of spread) 3. Distant metastases (M) or MX-Distant metastases can not be assessed (some doctors rarely use this name) or M0-No distant metastases or M1-Distant metastases are present As a consequence, a person's cancer may be labeled as T1N2M0, indicating that it is a tiny tumor (T1) which has spread to certain area lymph nodes (N2) and has no distant metastases (M0).

Of example, certain cancer registries use screening, epidemiology, and a descriptive staging system (SEER). SEER divides cancer patients into five major categories:

- In situ: irregular cells are found only in the layer of cells through which they have formed.

- Localized: Cancer is confined to the organ in which it started, without any signs of propagation.

- Regional: Cancer has spread to local lymph nodes, organs and tissues outside the main location.

- Remote: Cancer has spread from the main location to remote organs or to distant lymph nodes.

- Unknown: there is not enough details available to decide the point.

The diagnosis of cancer is important; it allows the surgeon to settle about the most appropriate treatment strategies, offers a framework for predicting the prognosis (outcome) for the individual, and offers a mechanism for transmitting the status of the individual to all health providers interested with medical care.

CHAPTER FIVE
WAYS TO EAT TO DEFEAT CANCER TODAY AND EVERY DAY

A big reason for cancer to be so frustratingly difficult to eradicate is that it is always very advanced and, like many chronic illnesses, far more challenging to handle by the time it can be diagnosed. For an advanced cancer patient, unchecked angiogenesis prevents cancer cells expanding and causes them to spread.

Nevertheless, without angiogenesis, cancers can not develop and become harmful. This is why microscopic cancers, which develop in our bodies all the time, are often harmless. These cancers are not often noticeable on a regular X-ray or body scan.

And, in order to combat cancer successfully, angiogenesis has to be managed until the tumor can gain a foothold. That is where the regular food falls into action.

Start Eating to Beat Cancer Today Feeding to Beat Cancer can be done by easily introducing a few cancer-fighting angio foods to your diet every day.

As life itself, one lifestyle is mostly about creating decisions. As we all eat every day, why not pick food that will reduce the risk of disease?

Disturbing recent work reveals that microscopic cancer, miniature cancer cells that can only be identified under a microscope, is common. A new survey of women in the 40s revealed that 40% of them have microscopic breast cancer. Perhaps more surprising is that nearly 100 percent of men in the 1970s would have small cancer in their thyroid glands.

A microscopic tumor will develop up to 16,000 times its original size in as little as two weeks. But the Angiogenesis Foundation's latest pioneering work shows that you will avoid cancer until it starts to spread. A modern therapeutic strategy is called angiogenesis.

Anti-angiogenesis allows you to improve your "social climate" by modifying the food you feed, thereby depriving cancer cells of the ability to develop and spread.

Some products, consumed with the right portion and amount, may have cancer-causing benefits. Below are the foods to be consumed that will keep cancer from growing:

1. Be Picky.

Red Delicious and Granny Smith apples produce half as many cancer survivors as Fuji and Golden Delicious apples.

The tomato produces more cancer fighter than any other type.

Wine grapes produced in colder temperatures produce more cancer-fighters than grapes produced in hot climates.

Apples, tomatoes and grapes on the Dirty Twelve list of the most pesticides released by the Environmental Working Group, and you can purchase organic goods if possible.

2. Eat the sprouts.

Broccoli sprout plate can have more cancer-fighting properties than normal broccoli.

3. Dunk Your Tea Cup

Dunking a tea bag up and down produces more cancer-fighting molecules than simply making the bag stay in the cup.

4. Cook tomatoes, please.

Fresh tomatoes are fine, but it's best to cook them in olive oil.

Editor's note: it is not appropriate to cook tomatoes in olive oil in order to enjoy the benefits. Nevertheless, cooking tomatoes increase the lycopene content and increase the cancer-fighting capacity. Lycopene is also a fat-soluble antioxidant, which means that it is easily processed by the body when eaten with any (ideally healthy) food.

5. Chew the Vegetables.

Chewing leafy greens helps trigger enzymes that enable cancer-fighting molecules deep in the trees.

6. Go to Soy.

Fermented soy, like the kind used in miso soup, produces four times as many cancer fighters as normal soybeans.

See why the research clearly shows that not only does soy not encourage cancer, but that John Robbins reduces the likelihood of cancer in this post. It is necessary to use organic soy products to avoid genetically modified soy. Some fermented soy products include tempeh and natto.

7. Select a Cancer-Fighting Food for every meal.

With three meals a day, more than a thousand cancer-fighting dietary options are introduced last year.

Without consuming the correct diets, cancer cells are starving to death because they do not have the blood supplies they need to live.

Bok Choy: This form of Chinese cabbage produces brassinin; a potent cancer-fighter often contained in broccoli, cauliflower and Brussels sprouts. Bok Choy can be consumed 3 days a week in 1/2 cup of servings to reap the maximum benefits.

Cooked tomatoes contain more cancer-causing agents than untreated tomatoes. Both produce lycopene, so the heating of the tomato shifts the chemical composition and allows the effects more readily accessible to the body. You will eat 2-3 (1/2 cup) servings of cooked tomatoes every week.

The species is high in omega-3 fatty acids and poor in mercury. It's perfect for three 6-ounce portions a week.

Strawberries The antioxidants in this berry help combat cancer. You will eat 1 cup of juice a day.

Artichokes carry three separate cancer-fighting molecules. Live 1/4 cup with hearts a day.

Can food help us starve cancer

Can we eat in order to starve cancer?

The reaction here is a resounding yes! What we consume is incredibly important when it comes to stopping and beating cancer.

However, in a society where statements on what can and does not raise our likelihood of contracting those cancers are sometimes contradictory, it is understandable that many can remain dubious regarding the argument that our body's natural protection mechanisms may be improved by the food we consume.

For this question, the theory of how we evolve up, how our DNA (our genes) manifest themselves in our up, how cells mutate and form clusters, and how these microscopic clusters advance into observable cancer. Once we realize how cells function and how various foods can either prevent or trigger the growth of cancer cells, the role that diet plays in keeping us alive starts to make a lot of sense.

With that in mind, I'm going to explain to you about a physiological cycle called angiogenesis.

But what is angiogenesis and what does it have to do with malnutrition cancer?

Angiogenesis is a mechanism used by our bodies to develop and sustain blood vessels. Under regular conditions, blood vessels sustain life, supplying oxygen and essential nutrients to all of our organs. Yet as dysfunctional blood vessels develop, microscopic cancers may be nourished. A stable angiogenesis mechanism controls when and where blood vessels are to develop and may discourage tumors from exploiting private blood sources for the oxygen they need to spread. If the body lacks its ability to regulate blood vessels, a broad variety of diseases, including cancer, can occur.

As long as the angiogenesis mechanism works correctly, the

blood vessels expand in the right location at the right time —
not too many, not too few, but just the right number. Holding a
optimal equilibrium of the circulatory system is at the root of
how angiogenesis preserves us by maintaining us in a
condition called homeostasis. Homeostasis is characterized as
preserving regular function equilibrium in the body when
adapting to continuously changing conditions. Angiogenesis
plays a crucial part in developing and preserving the whole
circulatory system and adjusting it to various circumstances in
our lives to preserve our health.

Because of this effective health protection mechanism, which
actually decreases the blood flow to tumors, cancer does not
have to be a disease.

If you don't believe you're at risk of getting cancer, so why
does it matter to you?

Okay, you would be shocked to hear that we all develop
microscopic cancers in our body all the time. Autopsy tests on
individuals who died in traffic crashes have found that
approximately 40 percent on women between the ages of 40
and 50 currently have tiny breast cancers. About 50 percent of
people in their 50s and 60s have microscopic prostate cancers,
and nearly 100 percent of us, by the time we enter our 70s,
would have microscopic cancers rising in our thyroid gland.

Yet without a blood stream, most of these cancers would never
become harmful. The capacity of the body to regulate
angiogenesis stops blood vessels from feeding tumors, so that
turned out to be one of our most significant cancer protection
mechanisms. In reality, if you block angiogenesis and prevent
blood vessels from entering cancer cells, the tumors literally

can not expand.

And, since angiogenesis is a turning point between healthy and dangerous cancer, a novel solution to cancer treatment is to cut off the blood flow by eating anti-angiogenic products.

It is discovered a variety of tasty foods (and beverages) that are actually anti-angiogenic: foods that can obstruct the development of blood vessels and, consequently, discourage cancer cells from ever growing into cancer, including among those among whom cancers are in the family.

For example, repeated studies have shown that the excess of fruits, plants, vegetables and spices, such as berries, grapes, soybeans, garlic and parsley, inhibits angiogenesis by more than 60%. Perhaps more interestingly, studies have found that variations of such foods supply our bodies with a more effective inhibitor of cancer than other other, which shows the beneficial influence of "other synergy" (eating a variety of nutritious foods rather than a lot of the same thing).

Understanding angiogenesis helps one to consider how we can continue to maintain ourselves stable and illness-free, and how we can possibly counteract the negative health consequences of inherited predisposition to illness or inadequate nutrition. Angiogenesis is a modern theory about how the body repairs itself, and the science's point is that our health effects are not predestined. We will combat illness by the food we consume.

Certain Foods May Increase Cancer Risk

It is difficult to prove that certain foods cause cancer.

However, observational studies have repeatedly shown that consuming certain foods in large amounts may increase the likelihood of cancer.

Sugar and refined carbohydrates

Processed foods high in sugar, low in fiber and nutrients are associated with a higher risk of cancer.

In particular, researchers have found that diets that cause blood sugar levels to rise are associated with an increased risk of various cancers, including stomach cancer, breast cancer, and colorectal cancer. A study of more than 47,000 adults found that people who eat a high-carbohydrate diet are almost twice as likely to die from colon cancer as people who eat a low-carb diet.

It is believed that higher blood sugar and insulin levels are carcinogenic factors. Insulin has been shown to stimulate cell division, support the growth and spread of cancer cells and make them more difficult to eliminate

In addition, higher insulin and blood sugar levels may cause inflammation in the body. In the long run, this may lead to abnormal cell growth and may lead to cancer.

This may be why people with diabetes (a disease characterized by high blood sugar and high insulin levels) have an increased risk of certain types of cancer.

For example, if you have diabetes, your risk of colorectal cancer is 22% higher.

To prevent cancer, limit or avoid foods that increase insulin levels, such as foods high in sugar and refined carbohydrates.

Processed meat products

The International Agency for Research on Cancer (IARC) believes that processed meat is a carcinogen that can cause cancer.

Processed meat refers to meat that has been cured, cured or smoked to maintain flavor. It includes hot dogs, ham, bacon, sausages, sausages and some deli meats.

Observational studies have found an association between consumption of processed meat and increased risk of cancer (especially colorectal cancer).

A large number of studies have found that people who consume large amounts of processed meat have an increased risk of colorectal cancer by 20% to 50% compared to those who rarely or not eat this food at all.

Another review involving more than 800 studies found that eating only 50 grams of processed meat a day-about four slices of bacon or a hot dog-increased the risk of colorectal cancer by 18%.

Some observational studies have also linked eating red meat to an increased risk of cancer. However, these studies usually do not distinguish between processed meat and unprocessed red meat, which can distort the results.

Multiple reviews combined the results of multiple studies and found that the evidence linking unprocessed red meat to cancer is weak and inconsistent

Cooked food

Cooking certain foods at high temperatures, such as grilling, frying, frying, grilling and grilling, can produce harmful compounds such as heterocyclic amines (HA) and advanced saccharification end products (AGEs)

Excessive accumulation of these harmful compounds can cause inflammation and may play a role in the development of cancer and other diseases

Certain foods, such as high-fat and high-protein animal foods, and highly processed foods, are most likely to produce these harmful compounds at high temperatures.

These include meat-especially red meat-certain cheeses, omelettes, butter, margarine, cream cheese, mayonnaise, oil and nuts.

To minimize the risk of cancer, avoid burning food and choose a milder cooking method, especially when cooking meat, such as steaming, stewing or boiling. Marinated foods also help.

Dairy

Several observational studies have shown that consuming a large amount of dairy products may increase the risk of prostate cancer

A study tracked nearly 4,000 men with prostate cancer. The results show that high intake of whole milk increases the risk of disease progression and death.

More research is needed to determine possible causality.

The theory suggests that these findings are due to increased intake of calcium, insulin-like growth factor 1 (IGF-1) or estrogen in pregnant cows-all of which are weakly linked to prostate cancer

Eating foods rich in sugar and refined carbohydrates as well as processed and cooked meat may increase the risk of cancer. In addition, higher consumption of dairy products is associated with prostate cancer.

Certain Foods Contain Cancer-Fighting Properties

There is no one super food worthy of stopping cancer. Instead, a balanced approach to eating is expected to be more effective.

Experts say that consuming an ideal cancer diet will reduce the chances by up to 70% and will possibly help you heal from cancer. Researchers also agree that other diets will combat cancer by restricting blood arteries that fuel cancer in a cycle called anti-angiogenesis.

Nevertheless, nutrition is complicated and the efficacy of such products in the battle against cancer differs based on whether they are produced, handled, stored and cooked.

Many of the main anti-cancer food classes include: Vegetables Observational studies have associated higher intake of vegetables with lower cancer risk. Most vegetables produce antioxidants and phytochemicals that combat cancer.

For starters, cruciferous vegetables, including broccoli, cauliflower and cabbage, include sulforaphane, a compound that has been shown to decrease tumor size in mice by more than 50% Certain vegetables, such as tomatoes and carrots, are correlated with reduced risk of prostate, stomach and lung cancer Fruit Similar to vegetables, fruits containing antioxidants and other phytochemicals,

One analysis showed that at least three servings of citrus fruit a week decreased the incidence of stomach cancer by 28 a cent of flaxseeds Flaxseeds have been correlated with preventive benefits against some cancers and can also minimize the spread of cancer cells For example, one research reported that people with prostate cancer had 30 grams — or around 4 1/4 tablespoons — of ground flaxseed regular experience. Similar effects have been observed in women with breast cancer

Spices

Certain test tubes and animal tests have shown that cinnamon could have anti-cancer properties and avoid the spread of cancer cells. In addition, curcumin, which is present in the turmeric, can help combat cancer. A 30-day study showed that 4 grams of curcumin daily decreased potentially cancerous lesions in the colon by 40 per cent in 44 non-treatment patients

Beans and Legumes

Beans and legumes are rich in fiber, and some studies indicate that higher intake of this nutrient can protect against colorectal cancer. One research of more than 3,500 people showed that those who eat the most legumes have up to a 50% reduced chance of those forms of cancer.

Nuts

Regularly consuming nuts can be correlated with a decreased risk of other forms of cancer For example, one analysis of more than 19,000 people showed that someone who consumed more nuts have a reduced chance of dying from cancer Olive Oil Several tests indicate a correlation between olive oil and a reduced risk of cancer.

A broad analysis of the retrospective trials showed that those who ate the largest volume of olive oil had a 42% reduced chance of cancer relative to the control group.

Garlic

Garlic produces allicin, which has been found to have cancer-fighting effects in test tube tests.

Certain reports also shown an correlation between the consumption of garlic and a reduced incidence of different forms of cancer, including stomach and prostate cancer

Fish

There is proof that consuming fresh fish can help defend against cancer, likely owing to healthier fats that may minimize inflammation.

A broad study of 41 research showed that consuming fish daily decreased the chance of colorectal cancer by 12%.

Dairy Some research indicates that consuming some dairy products can reduce the risk of colorectal cancer.

The form and quantity of milk consumed are significant.

Of starters, moderate intake of high-quality dairy goods, such as raw milk, fermented milk goods and grass-fed cow milk, can have a protective impact.

It is mostly attributed to elevated amounts of protective fatty acids, conjugate linoleic acid and fat-soluble vitamins. On the other side, high intake of mass-produced and refined dairy foods is correlated with an elevated risk of some diseases, including cancer. The causes for these effects are not well known, but could be related to hormones found in pregnant cow milk or IGF-1.

Being Overweight or Obese Is Linked to Increased Cancer Risk

Aside from smoking and hepatitis, obesity is the single largest risk factor for cancer worldwide.

This raises the chances of 13 specific forms of cancer, including esophagus, lung, pancreas, and kidney cancer, as well as menopausal breast cancer.

Across the US, weight issues are projected to blame for 14 per cent to 20 per cent of all cancer deaths of both men and women.

Obesity can raise the likelihood of cancer in three main ways:

- Excess body fat can lead to insulin resistance. As a consequence, the cells are unable to consume glucose adequately, which causes them to split more rapidly.

- Obese individuals continue to have elevated rates of

inflammatory cytokines in their plasma, which induces systemic inflammation and promotes cell division.

- Fat cells lead to higher estrogen rates, which raise the likelihood of breast and ovarian cancer in postmenopausal women. Great news is that multiple reports have found that weight reduction in overweight and obese individuals is expected to decrease the incidence of cancer. Overweight or obesity is one of the main risk factors for many forms of cancer. Achieving healthier weight will help guard against the risk of cancer.

Cancer and Fasting / Calorie Restriction

Will fasting or calorie restriction aid my body to battle cancer? Can it also help to render cancer care more effective?

Claim: Fasting and calorie restriction (CR) will delay and even halt cancer growth, destroy cancer cells, strengthen the immune system, and greatly increase the efficacy of chemotherapy and radiation therapy.

What's that?

First, let's describe CR versus fasting and discuss the past of these two activities. Calorie restriction involves restricting the intake of calories, without inducing starvation, to less than what an individual might consume if free access was given. Fasting, on the other side, is not able to consume any meal for different periods of time. Fasting has been seen as a cure for several medical illnesses as well as a form of spiritual /

religious activity throughout history.

Calorie Restriction: 20-40 per cent restriction of calorie consumption for a long period of time (1200 calories for women versus 1400 calories for men a day) Intermittent Calorie Restriction: 50-70 a cent restriction of calorie intake for a limited period of time (600-1000 calories a day) Fasting: total removal of calorie intake from 1 day to several weeks Intermittent fasting: Across centuries, several prominent doctors and several of the oldest therapeutic methods have advocated fasting as an important form of therapeutic and prevention. Hippocrates argued that fasting helped the body to repair itself.

Fasting is part of several of the world's faith practices, including Christianity, Hinduism, Judaism, Buddhism, and Islam. Some of the great spiritual figures in humanity fasted for intellectual and moral insight, like Christ, Buddha, and Mohammed. During one of the most well-known revolutionary activities of the past century, Indian leader Mahatma Gandhi fasted for 21 days to encourage harmony.

People have endured several lengthy stretches of drought throughout their existence, and while it is affected by several causes, it seems that most people will live on water alone for more than a month. Historically, most species have evolved in fluctuating food-availability conditions, during which time cycles of malnutrition were frequently observed, and selection has been selected for species capable of withstanding malnutrition.

What is the proof of that?

More than 100 years of work have been done into the function of calorie restriction in the likelihood of prolonging life. Although much of this work has been performed on livestock, a small amount of human knowledge has accrued which suggests a protective impact against secondary ageing. Furthermore, risk factors for atherosclerosis and diabetes are substantially decreased in humans following CR, along with inflammatory receptors such as C-reactive protein (CRP) and tumor necrosis factor (TNF) (Holloszy). We're going to dig into work directly on calorie control, fasting and disease. We can begin by looking at the physiological processes being investigated and then go on to investigate some fascinating human experiments.

Biology The response to hunger allows an individual to redirect resources to several defense mechanisms to mitigate harm that would impair health. It is believed that such devices will also extend life and reduce the incidence of cancer. CR without starvation is the most effective and reproducible biochemical action to improve lifespan and guard against cancer in mammals. CR decreases rates of anabolic hormones, growth factors and inflammatory cytokines, lowers oxidative stress and cell proliferation, improves autophagia (cell destruction) and other DNA repair processes One of the main metabolic factors in the above category is insulin-like growth factor-1 (IGF-1). We address the role of IGF-1 and cancer in the Sugar and Low Carbohydrate Diet pages of this website. An important finding made by Dr. Longo is that CR was only effective in lowering IGF-1 while protein consumption was not reduced. Increased protein consumption or healthy nitrogen balance has been correlated with decreased IGF-1. This is an significant observation, because many cancer patients are advised to raise their protein consumption through treatment; this advice will need to be revised.

There are a variety of issues with CR. Another is that it requires weeks, or even months, to be successful in making the physiological improvements mentioned above. Another problem is that it usually ends in a permanent reduction of weight. At least 15% weight reduction is predicted with modest (20 percent) CR. It could be good for those who are overweight, but for someone with a healthier weight or those who are only at a normal weight, it might contribute to underweight and undernourishment.

One alternative instead for CR might be sporadic CR or intermittent fasting, which might potentially be more safe and less weight-loss. This can result in increased declines in fat concentration, IGF-1, and cell proliferation, thus increasing the responsiveness of insulin and adiponectin. These findings come from early observations of random mammary tumor models on rodents, which contrasted fasting on alternating days vs fasting for 2-3 days per week. Both methods decrease the occurrence of tumors by 40-80 per cent relative to ad lib in a variety of studies, but the results of alternate-day intermittent fasting were more apparent.

There are three metabolic phases during starvation or fasting of carbohydrates. The first step will last 10 or more hours and utilizes glycogen stores for energy. When the glycogen reserves have been depleted, the body transforms into glycerol and free fatty acids produced from the adipose tissue. Such nutrients produce ketones that the body and brain will then use for energy. This process can last for several weeks, depending on the size and health of the individual.

In addition to fasting, a ketogenic diet, as defined in our Low Carbohydrate Diet portion, may also transform the energy source from glucose to fatty acids. Theoretically, ketogenic diets may be maintained for longer, as calories and other vital foods tend to be absorbed, while certain people can consider it challenging to manage diets. Through fasting, until the fat stores are depleted, muscle degradation continues to start to drive gluconeogenesis.

Like CR, fasting causes improvements in cellular defenses to defend against initial weight loss and improves defense against oxidative stress. Fasting results in a more substantial decrease in insulin rates as well as an rise in insulin responsiveness in a shorter span of time relative to CR. Given that insulin rates play a role in the prevention of cancer, these variations are potentially clinically significant.

It is further suggested that cancer cells do not respond to fasting-generated defensive signals, rendering them resistant to both the immune system and cancer care. This method is referred to as differential stress resistance (DSR). Short-term starvation (STS), fasting for 48 hours, triggers a rapid transition of cells to a defensive state, capable of shielding mammalian cells and mice from numerous poisons, including chemotherapy.

Science Studies The first research paper to note that CR prevented the development of transplanted tumors in mice was reported. Since then, a broad body of research has demonstrated that CR inhibits the growth of tumors in different animal models. More work in both mice and monkeys has found that while CR was begun at 12 months of age, lifespan improved and the occurrence of sporadic cancer decreased by 50 per cent. While most cancer cells do tend to be susceptible to CR, there are certain cells that bear mutations that render them immune to CR. This indicates that the potency of CR might be restricted to other forms of cancer. Human trials have been minimal to date; however, there are several important results linked to the reduction of cancer incidence and the reduction of treatment-based side effects.

Risk Reduction and Tumor Regression

In 2014, Longo and colleagues showed that fasting triggered the death of "dead" immune cells in mice, which were replaced by stem cells as soon as the subjects began eating again. We concluded that a 3-day rapid could help to restore a healthy immune system. Researchers also showed that 48-hour accelerated growth in mice delayed the progression of five of the eight cancers tested. The application of fasting periods with chemotherapy was found to be more successful than chemotherapy alone in all cancers treated (6). Since these were all experimental experiments, it is not clear if humans will have the same benefit; nevertheless, some successful clinical trials are investigating the impact of calorie restriction or fasting on cancer.

A 2007 study (n=16) showed that alternate- fasting, where one day calories remained at 400 for women and 600 for men, and the other day was unregulated, reduced blood glucose, insulin and IGF-1 levels, with long- risk reductions for chronic diseases, including cancer, diabetes and cardiovascular disease. Two calorie restriction trials, one involving people at significantly elevated risk of breast cancer (n=19) and the other involving newly diagnosed patients with pancreatic cancer (n=19), reported a reduction in serum markers (IGF, stearoyl-CoA desaturase, fatty acid desaturase, and aldolase C), likely linked to cancer risk and prognosis A recent analysis examined evidence from Women's Healthy. The suggested explanation for this finding is assumed to be related to improved glycemic regulation resulting in defense against carcinogenesis. Increasing 2-hour rise in nighttime fasting was correlated with a steadily lower degree of hemoglobin A1C. This work is especially important as it is a food technique that most people will follow.

Treatment Protection-Related Side Effects Fasting can often shield patients against adverse side effects of chemotherapy or radiation therapy. Fasting for up to five days, accompanied by a regular diet prior to treatment, can minimize the side effects of treatment without triggering excessive weight loss or interfering with the therapeutic impact of treatment. Elderly cancer patients (n=10) who spontaneously experienced short-term fasting before and/or after chemotherapy showed less side effects. A limited sample (n=6) recorded a decrease in nausea, exhaustion, and gastrointestinal side effects relative to fast-free chemotherapy, and a decline in several other side effects was also documented in a community of patients who were still fasting before chemotherapy.

Health In a broad longitudinal sample of 2000 people, fasting (350 kcal / day) was found to be healthy and helpful to their chronic illness (rheumatic disorders, chronic pain syndrome, asthma, metabolic syndrome). The main concern with calorie restriction and fasting as it relates to cancer is weight loss. When discussed earlier, weight reduction is generally less of a problem with short-term fasting than with long-term calorie limits. It can be a good side effect for those who are overweight; but, for cancer patients who are either underweight or unable to control their weight, further weight loss can be harmful and can be a contraindication to fasting or CR. This is also worth noting that side effects, such as fatigue, light-headedness, nausea or exhaustion, can arise while fasting for more than a few days. Side effects, such as anemia or amenorrhea, can arise with a fasting duration of many weeks. The longer it lasts, the more necessary it becomes to take control of the re-feeding. Every process has to be slow and continuous in order to avoid major complications – or even mortality – from arising out of a extended period of time.

Which is the recommendation?

Comparing studies between CR and fasting, fasting tends to show more positive effects and preserve healthy cells without the possibility of weight loss or immune suppression. All CR and Fasting are the focus of active experiments, and the findings of these trials are pending final conclusions. As described above, it might not be suitable for all, particularly those who are underweight or extremely sick, and should never be attempted without the guidance of trained practitioners.

For general cancer prevention, it could be helpful to incorporate occasional or short-term rapids in conjunction with a plant-based cancer prevention diet, as outlined in depth in the Dietary Strategies section of this website.

Here are few suggestions for bringing home from the review:

1. In general, eat an anti-inflammatory diet of plenty of

vibrant berries, fruits, grains, lentils, herbs and spices.

2. Small to moderate consumption of carbohydrate and reduced glycemic starches 3. Good fats for a meal, like healthy sources of Omega-3s 4. Low protein consumption of 3-4 oz. per meal from a mixture of animal and plant proteins 5. Lengthen the time between dinner and breakfast to make for a longer nighttime easy, with a goal of 13 or more hours, e.g. dinner by 6:00 p.m. and breakfast by 7:00 a.m.

1. 6. Short-term water levels of 1-3 days to aid potentially rebuild the immune system and improve cell defense against oxidative stress. Together alongside a healthcare professional, you will decide how much it would be necessary for you to get involved rapidly.

2. 7. When you are a cancer patient, water fasting 2-3 days before and up to one day after surgery can be recommended in order to improve the effectiveness of care and the medication-related side effects, but only under the guidance of a professional physician.

CHAPTER SIX
IMMUNE SYSTEM

The immune system is a complex cell and organ network that defends the organism from foreign biological effects. (Although in a wide context, nearly any organ has a defensive role, such as close seals of the skin or the acidic atmosphere of the stomach.) While the immune system is working correctly, it defends the body from microbes and viral diseases, killing cancer cells and foreign substances.

If the immune system weakens, its ability to defend the body also weakens, allowing pathogens, including viruses that cause common colds and flu, to grow and thrive in the body.

The immune system also monitors tumor cells, and immune suppression has been reported to increase the risk of certain types of cancer.

The immune system is a host protection mechanism that involves multiple biological mechanisms and processes within an individual that defends against disease. In order to work properly, the immune system must identify and differentiate a broad variety of organisms, recognized as pathogens, from viruses to parasitic worms, from the body's own healthy tissue. There are two main immune system subsystems of several species: the innate immune system and the adaptive immune system. Both subsystems use humoral immunity and cell-mediated immunity to perform their function. In humans, blood – brain barrier, blood – cerebrospinal fluid barrier, and related fluid – brain barriers distinguish the peripheral immune system from the neuroimmune system that protects the brain.

Pathogens can evolve and adapt quickly, avoiding detection and neutralization of the immune system; however, multiple defense mechanisms have also evolved to recognize and neutralize pathogens. Also basic unicellular species, such as bacteria, have a primitive immune system in the form of enzymes that guard against bacteriophage infections. Many essential immune systems also developed in ancient eukaryotes and survive in their current descendants, such as plants and invertebrates. These pathways include phagocytosis, antimicrobial peptides called defensins, and the complementary network. Jawed vertebrates, including humans, have even more sophisticated defense mechanisms, including the ability to adapt over time to better recognize specific pathogens. Adaptive (or acquired) immunity creates immunological memory after an initial response to a specific pathogen, resulting in an enhanced response to subsequent encounters with the same pathogen. This process of immunity is the basis of vaccination.

Immune system disorders can lead to autoimmune diseases, inflammatory diseases and cancer. Immunodeficiency occurs when the immune system is less active than normal, resulting in recurrent and life-threatening infections. In humans, immunodeficiency may be either the result of a genetic disease such as severe combined immunodeficiency, acquired conditions such as HIV / AIDS, or the use of immunosuppressive drugs. Autoimmunity, on the other hand, stems from a hyperactive immune system that targets human tissues as though they were alien species. Common autoimmune diseases include Hashimoto thyroiditis, rheumatoid arthritis, type 1 diabetes mellitus, and systemic lupus erythematosus. Immunology is concerned with studying all aspects of the immune system.

How self-reactive immune cells are allowed to develop

Shortly after conception, the immune system begins the development of a subtype of antibody-producing immune cells, B-1, which can survive for a lifetime. After that stage, no more B1-cells are produced. However, these cells are self-reactive — they not only generate antibodies to foreign substances, but also to the body's own substances, so it is not known that the immune system requires such individual cells to grow. The study team at Lund University in Sweden has now established a pathway to regulate the development of B1-cells in mice. The results, which can contribute to a greater understanding of some causes of cancer and autoimmune disorders, have recently been reported in Science Immunology.

B-1 cells are a self-reactive subset of B cells that constantly generate antibodies that may respond to the body's own substances. They are, therefore, helpful rather than detrimental, because there is also a need for poor self-reactivity to cope with dying or dead cells. B1-cells also continue to cleanse the blood, ensuring that there is no inflammation in the blood.

Previously, it was not known that the immune system might enable such unique self-reactive cells to remain. There are very stringent quality controls in the immune system that suppress certain self-reactive cells to avoid the production of autoimmune diseases.

"We have found a pathway in the form of a protein that enables the growth of B1-cells during the tightly controlled duration of the neonatal immune development in mice. Such B1-cells evolve during the prenatal stage and before two weeks after birth. After that, the protein is gone and the B1 cell development window is closed,"

The protein that makes this phase possible is Lin28b. When the protein is absent, the growth of B1-cells is disrupted, however if it is overexpressed, B1-cells often grow in adult mice.

"The adult immune system is thus comprised of a combination of freshly formed cells and cells that have evolved early in life and continue during life. We agree that immune cells have unique functions based on where they mature and defend the body in various ways. Long-lived immune cells bring with them memory of past interactions, meaning that all external exposures begin from the very beginning. The long-lived population of B1-cells is of vital significance for the life-long maintenance of the immune system and may lead to the control of autoimmune diseases and cancer.

"While studies have been performed on rodents, fascinating similarities have also been observed for humans, as B1-cell-like cells have been identified in umbilical cord blood. The next move is to consider how we can relate our findings to B-cell cancer and autoimmune diseases.

How cellular structure orchestrates immunologic memory

For every virus or vaccine, the memory cells type that the body utilizes to identify the pathogen. It has been understood for decades — but the nature of this cellular immunological memory has historically been difficult to pin down. Researchers at the University of Basel and the University Hospital Basel have now established a microanatomical area in memory cells that allows them to function rapidly in the first few hours of immune response, as stated in the journal Immunity.

The immune system of the human body recognizes pathogens that trigger illness and may respond more rapidly in case of repeated contact. Vaccines are a perfect illustration of how immunological knowledge can shield us from infectious diseases. In terms of function and effect, immunological memory is well understood — the individual remains healthy despite being exposed to the pathogen. However, the basic cellular mechanisms that enable immunological memory were previously unknown.

An international group of researchers led by Professor Christoph Hess of the Department of Biomedicine at the University of Basel and the University Hospital Basel have now developed a framework that is responsible for the rapid immunological memory of different immune cells (CD8 + memory T cells): these essential memory cells shape numerous associations between mitochondria — the cell-powered cells — and

Fast immune response

The fast immune memory reaction at these touch sites is simply "orchestrated," conclude the researchers. Memory cells accumulate all the signal delivery molecules and enzymes required for rapid immune reaction here — and are primed when the organism is again subjected to the disease-causing pathogen. This helps the body to easily shield itself from infection.

CHAPTER SEVEN
CANCER STARVATION THERAPY

Abnormal cell metabolism and excessive food consumption is one of the main biochemical features of cancers. As such, the technique of cancer deprivation therapy through restricting blood flow, depleting glucose / oxygen and other essential tumor nutrients has been extensively researched as an effective method to manage cancer. Nevertheless, some undesirable properties of such drugs, such as poor targeting effectiveness, undesired systemic side effects, increased tumor hypoxia, mediated drug tolerance, and increased risk of tumor metastases, restrict their potential usage. The latest production of starvation-nanotherapeutics coupled with other therapeutic approaches has demonstrated a positive ability to resolve the above disadvantages. A study addresses the latest developments in nano-therapeutic cancer starvation treatment and examines the obstacles and potential opportunities of these anti-cancer approaches.

Characterized by irregular cell proliferation and development at risk of metastases, cancer persists today a worldwide and lethal danger to human safety 1, 2. Throughout recent years, cancer deprivation treatment has developed as an efficient means of slowing tumor development and survival by preventing air flow or depriving their vital nutrients / oxygen supply 3-5. The transfer of nutrients may be prevented by blocking the blood flow of tumors with angiogenesis inhibiting agents (AIAs) 6, 7, vascular disrupting agents (VDAs), 8, 9 and transarterial chemoembolization agents (TACEs) 10. In addition, agents that can absorb intratumoral nutrients /

oxygen or mediate the absorption of important substances by tumor cells can often contribute to tumor malnutrition and necrosis 4, 5, 11, 12. Although some novel advantages have been seen in cancer therapy over the years, problems associated with such drugs, such as poor targeting effectiveness, elevated tumor hypoxia, acute coronary syndrome, impaired ventricular conduction, mediated drug resistance, and increased risk of tumor metastases, remain restricted in clinical applications 13-16.

Combination therapy using cancer deprivation agents with other cancer care methods has been found to be an efficient means of improving clinical effectiveness relative to the standard clinical procedure 17. Nevertheless, problems of free medicines, such as excessive ingestion of medications, low bioavailability and fast in vivo metabolism, have remained worried 18. Advances in micro / nanotechnology and cancer biology have stimulated the production of drug delivery systems for cancer treatment with improved effectiveness and minimal side effects 19-22. Between them, a number of nanomaterials focused on natural / synthetic polymers 23-29, liposomes 30, metal-organic frameworks (MOFs) 13, gold nanoparticles (NPs) 31 and silica NPs 11, 32, 33 have been used to co-deliver cancer-causing agents and other therapeutics with the goal of minimizing medication side effects 23, enhancing their target effectiveness 26, 27, through durability and half-life. In addition, a technique for cancer deprivation combined with multimodal nanomedicine has already been developed to accomplish synergistic cancer treatment, which has been proven to be an successful way to counteract the side effects of free drugs and result in superadditive therapeutic results 14, 15, 20.

There are two main pathways in the nature of starvation-nanotherapeutics. One is stopping / reducing the blood flow of the tumor by inhibiting / disrupting angiogenesis or specifically restricting the blood vessels 11, 23, 26, 36, 37. The other is depriving tumor cells of vital nutrients / oxygen supply by absorbing intratumoral nutrients / oxygen, or reducing the absorption of important nutrients 4, 38-40. To improve clinical effectiveness, these clinicians cooperated with other cancer management methods, including chemotherapy 41, 42, gene therapy 43, phototherapy 44, 45, gas therapy 46, and immunotherapy 47. Herein, we study the latest attempts to exploit nanomedicine-based drug delivery systems for cancer starvation therapy and concentrate on core approaches for multimodal synergistic starvation management. Both the conceptual criteria and the anti-cancer efficacy of these formulations are illustrated. At the end of the day, the problems and potential opportunities in this sector are addressed.

Antiangiogenesis-related cancer starvation therapy

Tumor development and metastases are strongly dependent on angiogenesis, which is the critical stage in neoplasms from benign to malignant transformation. Anti-angiogenic therapy is an important way to combat tumor development by inhibiting main angiogenic activators. After 2003, many AIAs have been licensed by the Food and Drug Administration (FDA) for clinical cancer care. However, the related toxicity of these AIAs is not available for the clinical / preclinical review, which involves hypertension, artery swelling, weakening of blood vessels and proteinuria.

Nano-antiangiogenesis-based cancer monotherapy Compared to free AIAs, nanomedicine could both increase their therapeutic outcomes through controlling their release activity and enhancing drug accumulation at the tumor site via improved permeability and retention (EPR) results, as well as actively targeting tumors and/or endothelial cells through surface conjugation with target ligands. For example, mesoporous silica nanoparticles (MSNs) may dramatically increase the targeting efficacy of tanshinone IIA (an angiogenesis inhibitor) to HIF-15-007 overexpression, leading to improved antiangiogenesis behavior in the mouse colon tumor model (HT-29).

Several over-expressed receptors, such as integrin 5-007vβ3 and Neuropilin-1, have been used as nanomedicine targets, which have demonstrated enhanced targeting effectiveness and increased tumor inhibition efficiency. In addition, paclitaxel (PTX) primed antiangiogenic polyglutamic acid (PGA)-PTX-E-[c(RGDfK)2] nanoscale conjugate has been shown to significantly reduce the development and spread of endothelial (EC)-expressing endothelial cells (ECs) and several cancer cells. In addition, bevacizumab, a vascular endothelial growth factor (VEGF) angiogenesis inhibitor, was specifically used as a targeting ligand for the modulation of magnetic iron oxide nanoparticles (IOPs), which has been shown to be an important vector for bevacizumab delivery in mice with breast tumor (4T1).

Nanonization techniques for AIAs may not only decrease their related toxicity and increase antitumor efficacy to some degree, but also include a multi-drug co-delivery mechanism to maximize AIAs-based combination anticancer efficacy.

Synergistic antiangiogenesis/chemotherapy

Angiogenesis antagonists have also been used along with chemotherapy to resolve their deficiencies and boost antitumor efficacy. Recently, forms of optimized anti-angiogenic nanotherapy have been developed for cancer combination therapy. For example, doxorubicin (DOX) and mitomycin C (MMC) co-charged polymer-lipid hybrid nanoparticles may dramatically improve animal survival and tumor recovery compared to liposomal DOX for the treatment of multidrug-resistant human mammary tumor xenografts.

DOX association with methotrexate (MTX), which was co-supplied with MSNs, may also greatly increase the effectiveness of oral squamous cell carcinoma treatment by reducing the level of the lymph dispersion factor (VEGF-C). Zhu and coworkers have synthesized the matrix metalloproteinase-2 (MMP-2)-responsive nanocarrier for co-delivery of camptothecin (CPT) and sorafenib, which has been shown to be an important route to colorectal cancer synergistic treatment. Curcumin (Cur), a powerful anti-angiogenesis agent, was co-charged with DOX in pH-responsive poly(beta-amino ester) copolymer NPs for 4T1 tumor therapy, which showed intense anti-angiogenic and pro-apoptotic action.

Synergistic antiangiogenesis/gene therapy

Co-delivery of anti-angiogenesis medications and gene silencing agents is known to be another successful method of managing cancer through malnutrition. For starters, Lima and coworkers synthesized chlorotoxin (CTX) conjugate liposomes for anti-miR-21 oligonucleotide transmission, which encouraged the effectiveness of miR-21 silencing and improved antitumor activity with less systemic immunogenicity. Liu et al. also observed that the fusion suicide gene (yCDglyTK) could induce tumor cell apoptosis more effectively after co-dispensing calcium phosphate nanoparticles (CPNPs) with VEGF siRNA, where the density of capillary vessels was also clearly decreased in gastric carcinoma xenograft tissue (SGC7901). In fact, poly-VEGF siRNA / thiolate-glycol chitosan nanocomplexes have been used to support Kim and coworkers solve the reactive issue of bevacizumab. The findings revealed that the combination of these two VEGF inhibitors induced synergistic effects with reduced VEGF expression and drug tolerance.

Synergistic antiangiogenesis/phototherapy

Nanomaterial-based phototherapy, which can specifically destroy cancer cells without usual tissue damage, has generated significant attention in cancer care. Enhanced antitumor activity was also shown when angiogenesis inhibitors and phototherapy agents were mixed. For eg, Kim and coworkers have established a hybrid RNAi-based AuNP nanoscale assembly (RNAi-AuNP) for combined anti-angiogenesis gene therapy and photothermal ablation, AuNPs changed by single-sense / anti-sense RNA sequences may be self-assembled into different geometric nanoconstructions (RNAi-AuNP).

The PEI / RNAi-AuNP complex was then prepared with branched polyethylene (BPEI) for successful intracellular transmission. Following intratumoral administration, the therapeutic effects of PEI / RNAi-AuNP complexes may be triggered by continuous wavelength lasers or high-intensity intense ultrasound, contributing to successful antiangiogenesis and tumor ablation. In another study, a carrier-free nanodrug was prepared by self-assembly of Sorafenib and chlorine e6 (Ce6) for antiangiogenesis and photodynamic therapy.

This nanodrug demonstrated strong passive targeting activity at tumor sites and successful in vivo reactive oxygen species (ROS) generation capability. Upon combination with Sorafenib, the rate of tumor inhibition was substantially increased. With additional benefits, such as strong biosafety and biocompatibility, this nano-integrated approach offered scope for cancer synergistic care in clinics.

CHAPTER EIGHT
VDAS-BASED CANCER STARVATION THERAPY

VDAs, as a unique class of anticancer compounds, is designed to selectively prevent the established abnormal tumor blood vasculature by targeting ECs and pericytes, leading to tumor starvation and central necrosis through hypoxia and nutrient deprivation. However, they are powerless to the cancer cells at the tumor margin, which could draw oxygen and nutrients from the surrounding normal tissues. Beside this, several other vascular risk factors, such as the acute coronary syndromes, blood pressure alteration, abnormal ventricular conduction, and transient flush, also limit the further application of free VDAs. To overcome the above issues and enhance their antitumor ability, VDAs-based multimodal cancer therapies have been developed for solid tumor treatments.

Free VDAs-enhanced nanomedicine-based chemotherapy

The barriers of heterogeneity and high interstitial fluid pressure of solid tumors not only limit the targeting efficiency of nanomedicines, but also weaken their antitumor ability against the tumor central area. Recent studies reported that small free molecule VDAs could help nanomedicines to overcome the above drawbacks. For example, Chen and coworkers developed a coadministration strategy using free CA4P and CDDP-loaded PLG-g-mPEG NPs (CDDP-NPs) for complementing each other's antitumor advantages and improving the antitumor efficiency. The multispectral optoacoustic tomography (MSOT) images indicated that the tumor penetration of CDDP-NPs highly relied on the tumor vasculature, which aggregated in the peripheral region of the tumors. While co-administration of free CA4P and CDDP-NPs improved the tumor cellular killing efficiency both in the central and peripheral regions according to hematoxylin and eosin (H&E) staining. The enhanced antitumor efficiency against both murine colon cancer (C26) and human breast cancer (MDA-MB-435) models supported that this combination strategy was a promising way for solid tumor treatment.

Furthermore, small molecule VDAs could induce tumor target amplification of ligand-coated NPs through selectively modifying tumor vasculature. For example, protein p32, a stress-related protein which is specifically expressed on the surface of tumor cells, can selectively bind with the phage-displayed cyclic peptide (LyP-1). Ombrabulin, a small molecule VDAs, was used to induce the local upgraded presentation of protein p32 for enhancing the tumor "active targeting" of LyP-1 coated NPs. The in vivo results demonstrated that the recruitment of LyP-1 coated DOX-loaded NPs significantly increased after pretreating with ombrabulin when compared with the control groups.

In another work, coagulation-targeted polypeptide-based NPs were developed for improving their tumor-targeting accumulation by homing to VDA-induced artificial coagulation environment. The in vivo results showed that this cooperative targeting system recruited over 7-fold higher CDDP doses to the tumors than non-cooperative control groups. The above cooperative targeting strategies combining with free VDAs and ligand-coated NPs showed obviously decreased tumor burden and prolonged mice survival compared to the non-cooperative controls.

VDAs-nanomedicine induced synergistic starvation/chemotherapy

VDAs-nanomedicine could enhance their accumulation and retention at the leaky tumor vasculature via EPR effect, leading to high distribution and gradual release of VDAs around the immature tumor blood vessels as well as prolonged vascular disruption effect compared to free drugs. Beside this, nanomedicine also provides a platform for VDAs-based cancer multimodal therapy.

For instance, a multi-compartmental "nanocell" integrating a DOX-PLGA conjugate core and a phospholipid shell was prepared for achieving temporal release of DOX and combretastatin A4 (CA4). After accumulating at the tumor site, CA4 was released from the outer phospholipid shell of the nanocell rapidly and attacked the tumor blood vessels, and DOX was then released subsequently from the inner polymeric core for killing tumor cells directly. This mechanism-based strategy exhibited reduced side toxicity and enhanced therapeutic synergism in the progress of inhibiting murine melanoma (B16F10) and Lewis lung carcinoma growth.

Furthermore, several polymer-VDA conjugates caused amplified TME characteristics was also utilized to develop new cancer co-administration strategies. Hypoxia is one of the major features of solid tumors which can promote neovascularization, drug resistance, cell invasion and tumor metastasis. Meanwhile, the existence of hypoxia also provides the desired target for tumor selective therapy. Tirapazamine (TPZ) is a typical hypoxia-activated prodrug (HAP), which own low toxicity toward normal tissues and can selectively kill the hypoxic cells after conversion into cytotoxic benzotriazinyl (BTZ) radical within hypoxic regions.

Nevertheless, the insufficient hypoxia level within tumors tremendously limited its further clinical application. To address this, Chen and coworkers proposed a cooperative strategy based on VDA-nanomedicine and HAPs for solid tumor treatment. In this study, poly(L-glutamic acid)-CA4 conjugate nanoparticles (CA4-NPs) were employed to selectively disrupt the abnormal vasculature of the tumor, as well as elevating the hypoxia level of the tumor microenvironment (TME). The intensive hypoxic TME further boosted the antitumor efficacy of TPZ subsequently. The in vivo results demonstrated that this combinational strategy can not only completely suppress the small tumor growth (initial tumor volume: 180 mm3), but also obviously keep down the size of large tumors (initial tumor volume: 500 mm3) without distal tumor metastasis.

Moreover, Chen and coworkers also demonstrated that the expression of matrix metalloproteinase 9 (MMP9, a typical tumor-associated enzyme) in treated tumors (4T1) could be markedly increased by more than 5-fold after treatment with CA4-NPs. These overexpressed MMP9 could further activate the DOX release from a MMP9-sensitive doxorubicin prodrug (MMP9-DOX-NPs) and enhance the in vivocooperative antitumor efficacy.

Vascular blockade-induced cancer starvation therapy

Besides the strategies of anti-angiogenic therapy and VDAs-induced tumor blood vessel disrupting, another promising strategy for cancer starvation therapy was proposed by shutting off the blood supply with nanothereapeutics that could selectively blockade tumor vascular and then inducing tumor necrosis.

Tumor-homing peptides-induced cancer starvation therapy

Tumor-homing peptides (THPs), such as pentapeptide (CREKA) and 9-amino acid cyclic peptide (CLT-1), could specially bind with fibrin-fibronectin complex in tumor blood clots. Based on this, Ruoslahti and coworkers developed a CREKA modified IONPs for fibrin-fibronectin complexes targeting and subtle clotting in tumor vessels. The initial deposition of these CREKA-IONPs created new binding sites for the subsequent NPs, and further enhanced the blood coagulation in the tumor lesion.

The results indicated that the tumor imaging efficiency of this self-amplifying tumor homing system owned about six-fold enhancement compared to the control groups. However, the tumor inhibition efficiency of this system showed no significant improvement due to the insufficient tumor vessel occlusion. To this end, a cooperative theranostic system containing CREKA-IONPs and CRKDKC-coated iron oxide nanoworms was further developed by the same research group for improving the clots binding efficacy. The results proved that this combination system led to 60~ 70% tumor blood blockades and obvious tumor size reduction in vivo.

Thrombin-mediated cancer starvation therapy

Thrombin is a serine protease that catalyzes series of coagulation-related reactions and leads to rapid thrombus formation during the clotting process. If thrombin can be precisely delivered to the tumor site and lead to selective occlusion of tumor-associated vessels by inducing the local blood coagulation, it might be a promising way for inhibiting the growth and metastasis of tumors. Recently, a nucleolin-targeting multifunctional DNA nanorobotic system was constructed for smart drug delivery. The presence of the nucleolin subsequently triggered the opening of these DNA nanotubes and released the loaded therapeutic thrombin, which then led to specific intravascular thrombosis and tumor vessel blockade at the tumor site. The growth of several tumor models was suppressed efficiently after treating with this thrombin-loaded DNA nanorobot, demonstrating that this system could become an attractive platform for cancer starvation therapy in a precise manner.

Deoxygenation agent-induced cancer starvation therapy

It is known that insufficient oxygen (O_2) supply could result in hypoxia-induced tumor cell necrosis. Based on this, Zhang et al. designed an injectable polyvinyl pyrrolidone (PVP)-modified magnesium silicide (Mg_2Si) nanoparticle as a nano-deoxygenation agent (nano-DOA) for directly consuming the intratumoral O_2 and starving tumors. This polymer-coated Mg_2Si NPs could respond to the slightly acidic TME after the intratumoral injection, and be converted into silicon dioxide (SiO_2) by scavenging the surrounding O_2 at the tumor site. As a byproduct, the in situ formed SiO_2 aggregates further occluded the tumor capillaries and obstructed the follow-up nutrient and O2 supply.

On the other hand, the intratumoral hypoxic level was also enhanced in the progress of O2 consuming with the presence of DOA. Given this reason, Bu and coworkers prepared a TPZ loaded PVP-modified Mg2Si nanoparticles (TPZ-MNPs) for drug delivery and combination cancer therapy. After intratumoral injection, the TPZ-MNPs quickly scavenged the O2 in situ and created an artificial anaerobic environment which caused the surrounding cell dormancy. Meanwhile, the released TPZ was activated in this promoted hypoxia TME, which further caused the now-dormant tumor cells death.

GOx-mediated cancer starvation therapy

Glucose is the major energy supplier for tumor growth and proliferation. Glucose oxidase (GOx) can specifically catalyze the conversion of glucose into gluconic acid and hydrogen peroxide (H2O2) with the involvement of O2. This reaction can directly consume glucose and O2, and elevate the local acidity, hypoxia and oxidation stress in vivo. Given this background, GOx has aroused considerable interest for cancer diagnosis and treatment in the past decade. Nevertheless, there are several limitations of this approach when using GOx as an anticancer agent. On the one hand, the overproduced H2O2 of glucose oxidation can cause systemic toxicity and lethal chain reactions through directly damaging cell membranes, proteins and DNA of normal cells. On the other hand, similar glucose supply and physiological requirement of normal cells often lead to off-targeting and ineffective starvation treatment. Through nanomedicine, GOx can co-delivery with other therapeutic agents for cancer multimodal treatments. Herein, we overview the recent representative GOx-based nanomedicines for cancer starvation therapy.

GOx-based cancer monotherapy

GOx could be used as an antitumor agent alone through consuming the intratumoral glucose and making the tumor "starving". The continuously generated H_2O_2 could further lead to DNA damage and tumor cell apoptosis. For example, Dinda et al. prepared a GOx-entrapped biotinylated vesicle for active targeting cancer starvation therapy. This GOx-containing system showed about six-fold higher tumor cell killing efficiency compared to normal cells through depleting the glucose supply for tumor cells in vitro.

However, the glucose depletion efficiency was restrained by the hypoxic TME in vivo, because of the insufficient O_2 supply in the solid tumor. Therefore, a hyaluronic acid (HA)-coated GOx and MnO_2 coloaded nanosystem (GOx-MnO_2@HA) was constructed for enhancing cancer starvation therapy outcome. After uptaking by the CD44-expressing tumor cells, the local glucose was converted into gluconic acid and H_2O_2 with GOx catalysis. The generated H_2O_2 then reacted with MnO_2 to generate O_2, which further accelerated the local glucose-consumption. This nanosystem provided benefit to break the hypoxia obstacles and enhance the antitumor effect by GOx.

Other strategies for cancer starvation therapy

Recently, types of special strategies in this field, which aimed at some critical nutrients, such as lactate and cholesterol, were also developed.

Lactate, which was once considered to be the waste product of glycolysis, has been demonstrated that can "fuel" the oxidative tumor cells growth as an energy substrate. Investigation indicated that interfering the lactate-fueled respiration could selectively kill the hypoxic tumor cells via inhibiting the expression of lactate-proton symporter, monocarboxylate transporter 1 (MCT1). Meanwhile, the reduction of lactate uptake by inhibiting the expression of MCT1 could transform the lactate-fueled aerobic respiration to anaerobic glycolysis as well as lower the O2 consumption in tumor cells which would facilitate the O2-depleting cancer therapy. For example, Zhang and coworkers developed an α-cyano-4-hydroxycinnamate (CHC) loaded porous Zr (IV)-based porphyrinic metal-organic framework (PZM) NPs with HA coating for cancer combination therapy.

After effectively accumulating at the CT26 tumors, the released CHC could obviously decrease the expression of MCT1 and turn down the lactate uptake which leading to lower the O2 consumption. As a result, the PDT efficiency was markedly enhanced due to the sufficient 3O2converting upon the laser irradiation (600 nm). Additionally, reducing the production of lactate via knockdown of lactate dehydrogenase A (LDHA) in tumor cells was also demonstrated that could neutralize of the tumor acidity and enhance the anti-PD-L1-mediated immunotherapy.

Recently, Thaxton and coworkers designed synthetic high density lipoprotein nanoparticles (HDL-NPs) with gold NPs as a size- and shape-restrictive template for lymphoma starvation therapy. This HDL-NPs could specially target scavenger receptor type B-1 (SR-B1), which is a high-affinity HDL receptor expressed by lymphoma cells. This combination of SR-B1 promoted the cellular cholesterol efflux and limited the cholesterol delivery, which selectively induced cholesterol starvation and cell apoptosis. The B-cell lymphoma growth was obviously inhibited after HDL-NPs treatment of B-cell lymphoma bearing mice.

Furthermore, this HDL-NPs could reduce the activity of myeloid-derived suppressor cells (MDSCs), a type of innate immune cells that potently inhibit T cells, through specifically binding with SR-B1of MDSCs. In Lewis lung carcinoma mice model, the in vivo data showed that the suppression of MDSCs by HDL-NPs markedly increased CD8+ T cells and reduced Treg cells in the metastatic TME. After treating with HDL-NPs, the tumor growth and metastatic tumor burden were obviously reduced and the survival rate was clearly improved due to enhanced adaptive immunity.

As an attractive strategy for cancer treatment, nanomedicine-mediated cancer starvation therapy could selectively deprive the nutrients and oxygen supply through antiangiogenesis treatment, tumor vascular disrupting or blockade, direct depletion of the intratumoral glucose and oxygen, and other processes. Moreover, by combining with chemotherapeutic drugs, therapeutic genes, enzymes, metal NPs, hypoxia-activated prodrugs, inorganic NPs, Fenton-reaction catalysts, photosensitizers, or photothermal agents, two or more therapeutic agents could be readily integrated into one single formulation, leading to enhanced treatment outcomes.

However, most innovations in this field are still in their infancy, with underlying challenges regarding clinical translation that need to be assessed in detail. For example, the biosafety of these nanomaterials is still significantly concerned, especially for the non-biodegradable formulations. Although the biosafety assessment of these materials could be systematically evaluated through animal models, long-term internal metabolic behaviors and related toxicity should be thoroughly investigated before clinical application. Another major concern is the aggravating hypoxia level that may accelerate the tumor invasion and metastasis in the progress of tumor starvation therapy.

Detailed studies should be performed to confirm whether cancer starvation therapy could turn on the tumor metastasis switch by elevating the hypoxic TME, which would also help to develop new combination strategies for offering synergistic effects. Moreover, in addition to elevating the hypoxia level, these cancer starvation-based methods could also increase the intratumoral acidity and/or promoting the intracellular oxidative stress. It remains unknown how these changes influence the local and systemic immune responses. The advances in cancer immunotherapy would offer new insights and perspectives for further evolving cancer starvation-based treatments

CHAPTER NINE
BEYOND SUGAR: WHAT CANCER CELLS NEED TO GROW

Amino acid glutamine is a lesser known nutrient on which cancer cells rely for development.

Cancer cells, like all cells, require nutrients to expand. Sugar is an essential power, but the only prerequisite for cancer is far from it. Present work focuses on cancer reliance on amino acid glutamine as a vulnerability.

In 1955, an American doctor called Harry Eagle made a shocking observation of cancer cells developing in a dish: they needed insane levels of glutamine. Without this chemical, the cells will stop developing and ultimately die, ignoring all the other recognized life requirements.

Glutamine is an amino acid, one of the 20 molecules that tie cells together into proteins. It is abundant in the nitrogen factor and can be broken down to supply the ingredient for the assembly of certain molecules, such as DNA.

Cancer cells addicted to glutamine have long been pursued by cancer biologists as a possible heel of Achilles for the management of the disease.

You learn even less about glutamine than you do about fructose, the other element that cancer cells prefer to absorb in excess. But it's just as necessary, though.

"Cells are so reliant on glutamine in so many respects, it is not only used in the processing of DNA nucleotides and other proteins, but it also serves as a money to compensate for the introduction of certain amino acids into the organism." Glutamine addiction to cancer cells has long attracted cancer biologists as a possible heel of Achilles to cure the disease. Maybe by cutting off the supply of this amino acid, cancer cells will starve to death. Inconveniently, regular cells do require glutamine. Drugs that reduce the amount of glutamine in the body are also considered dangerous to be used in cancer treatment.

But as scientists know more on how cancer cells utilize glutamine, they expect to discover new approaches to specifically kill cancer dependency while protecting regular cells.

Glutamine: An Essential Nonessential Amino Acid

In addition, the dependency of cancer on glutamine is quite startling. Technically, glutamine is a non-essential amino acid. Unlike important amino acids, which cells can not produce on their own and must receive from the food we consume, cells can quickly synthesize glutamine from other starting materials. Yet the many qualities of glutamine make it special.

"What is unique regarding glutamine is that all other non-essential amino acids may be derived from it, however certain non-essential amino acids can not substitute for glutamine. This is also crucial to many biochemical processes utilized by cancer cells to create new cell sections.

The cancer's requirement for glutamine is so high that certain cancer-causing oncogenes change how many the cells suck in and ingest. One of the best documented, the MYC gene, encourages cancer in part by growing cancer cells 'exposure to a constant supply of glutamine. Cells with an activated MYC gene allow some of the enzyme that transforms glutamine to its downstream components. Essentially, these cells are susceptible to MYC amplification.

Mutations in the IDH1 and IDH2 genes, which often affect the way glutamine compounds are used in cells, are widespread in some forms of brain cancer and leukemia.

The strong demand for glutamine implies that the amount of glutamine within the tumor is also very small. But cancer cells are already growing there. What is that?

This indicates that cells have alternate forms to replace their supply of glutamine. One such adaptation that she and her collaborators have observed is an improvement in the amount of the enzyme glutamine synthetase that produces glutamine from other starting materials, including glucose.

Her colleagues from the Thompson Lab and collaborators at Princeton University and New York University (NYU) have also shown that cancer cells can consume the cells surrounding them and scavenge their glutamine nutrients.

Targeted Deprivation

The adaptability of cancer cells to gain nutrients even though scarce allows any easy solution to cutting off the supply of cancer glutamine likely to fail.

There are, indeed, potential solutions. One is to directly inhibit the influx of glutamine into tumor cells. Some work shows that the protein transporter used by tumor cells to absorb glutamine is distinct from that used by regular cells, and that the transporter is more concentrated in tumor cells. Such cancer-specific transporters may be a strong choice for medications that will discourage the cells from meeting their remedy.

The reliance of cancer cells on glutamine may also act as a foundation for tailoring treatments of different people. Glutathione is a glutamine-dependent amino acid drug. Such essential cellular antioxidant dissolves toxic chemicals called reactive oxygen species and certain medications.

"Glutathione is bound to the medication and the kind of flags it needs to be separated from the tissue. Research by NYU scientists have shown that lung cancer tumors with some gene mutations are strongly reliant on glutathione. Interfering with their utilization (through medications named glutaminase inhibitors) may be a possible therapeutic strategy.

Some current clinical studies pair these glutamine-altering medications with immune checkpoint inhibitors or tyrosine kinase receptor signaling inhibitors, a big signal that signals cells to absorb and develop nutrients.

Just fat, just cancer, huh? A Look at the Proof A great deal has been published regarding the association between sugar and cancer. Much of that is incorrect.

Diagnostic Uses

In addition to the treatment choices, there are several screening tools. Just as glucose-loving cancer serves as the foundation for FDG-PET scans, its reliance on glutamine may serve as another useful diagnostic device. This will be especially beneficial for brain tumors. PET scans are less effective for detecting main brain cancers or cancers that have spread to the brain from somewhere else in the body as the brain itself uses up a lot of glucose. Glutamine-based scanning will enable doctors to tell cancer cells apart from regular brain cells.

No Dietary Solution

One solution to starvation glutamine cancer that is almost likely to fail is a shift of lifestyle. "We can't really change glutamine rates with food because the body appears to be doing such a decent job at maintaining the amount at a very stable concentration. The only time glutamine rates drops is through extreme pain or sepsis, which isn't anything you'd like to duplicate.

"At least for glucose, we might claim, 'Try to stop glucose spikes by consuming low glycemic products,' and so on, but with glutamine, it's a lot more challenging to create any practical suggestions.

CHAPTER TEN
STARVE CANCER CELLS
OF GLUTAMINE

Distinct from normal differentiated tissues, cancer cells reprogram nutrient intake and consumption to satisfy their strong demands for biosynthesis and energy output. The decreased usage and reliance on glutamine, a non-essential amino acid, for cancer cell growth and survival is a characteristic of these forms of reprogramming. It is well known that glutamine is a flexible biosynthetic substrate in cancer cells outside its function as proteinogenic amino acid.

In addition, growing data indicates that the synthesis of glutamine is controlled by several influences, including tumor background, oncogene / tumor suppression status, epigenetic alternation and tumor microenvironment. However, given the growing understanding of why cancer cells rely on glutamine for growth and survival, the role of glutamine metabolism to tumor development under physiological conditions is still under study, partially because glutamine levels in the tumor environment are still small.

As a current therapeutic approach for cancer has been developed to address the absorption and use of glutamine, learning how tumor cells react and responding to glutamine deficiency is key to improved therapeutic action. In this study, we first outline the broad usage of glutamine to promote cancer cell growth and survival, and then concentrate our debate on the effect of other nutrients on cancer cell tolerance to glutamine malnutrition, as well as its consequences for cancer therapy.

More than half a century ago, Harry Eagle found that supplementation of glutamine at millimolar rates in the tissue culture medium could improve cell growth and spread. By then, glutamine has become an important resource in most western tissue culture outlets. The rationale for the usage of exogenous glutamine, which is typically 5-to 20-fold higher than every other specific amino acid in tissue culture media, has only lately come into view as a consequence of tremendous advancement in the field of cancer cell metabolism. This is now well understood that glutamine is a flexible biosynthetic substrate for the supply of carbon and nitrogen atoms for the production of I m. These important precursors include nucleotides, non-essential amino acids (NEAAs) and fatty acids, which are basic building blocks for nucleic acids, proteins and lipids. In addition, glutamine or glutamine-derived metabolites may regulate energy supply, redox regulation, gene transcription and intracellular signaling. The inhibition of glutamine synthesis has also demonstrated therapeutic efficacy in pre-clinical settings by manipulating these growth-promoting processes.

In comparison to in vitro tissue culture environments under which glutamine is supplied at millimolar levels, the amount of glutamine under tumor tissues in vivo was observed to be slightly lower relative to standard surrounding tissues or plasma. Improved local intake of glutamine to promote tumor cell growth and low vascular supply are assumed to lead to the above findings. While these seminal experiments offered just a glimpse of the role of nutrients in the tumor system, they established the standard for studying tumor cells 'reactions to the restriction of glutamine. In comparison, the reduction of glutamine catabolism did not have a clinical advantage in certain tumor models.

Further analysis of the molecular mechanism used by tumor cells to respond to the restriction of glutamine will create avenues for understanding tumor development in a glutamine-limiting setting, or the reaction of tumor cells to therapies that inhibit the acquisition and/or use of glutamine. Throughout the past five years, evolving research has demonstrated that exposure to certain nutrients can affect the dependency of tumor cells on exogenous glutamine, allowing the identification of the most restrictive metabolite for tumor development during glutamine starvation. Throughout this study, we will address the impact of other NEAAs, including asparagine, aspartate, arginine and cystine, on the reliance of tumor cells on glutamine and their biological / therapeutic consequences.

Glutamine, a Versatile Biosynthetic Substrate

Glutamine is an NEAA that can be synthesized de novo with the use of glucose-derived carbon and free ammonia in mammals. Thus, the acquisition of glutamine through diet is not required. Even now, glutamine is one of the most common amino acids in human plasma (0.5~0.8 mM) associated with its flexible function as a biosynthetic substrate. Next, glutamine contains carbon and nitrogen atoms to synthesize nucleotides and other NEAAs. Carbon and nitrogen atoms may, of course, come directly from glutamine or glutamine-derived metabolites at several biosynthetic measures.

For illustration, during the synthesis of inosine monophosphate (IMP), a purine precursor, two nitrogen atoms are obtained from the Δ location of two glutamine molecules. The third nitrogen is provided by aspartate. Nonetheless, this nitrogen atom in aspartate is naturally extracted from glutamate by transamination; thus glutamate can be created from glutamine through a series of reactions that extract the nitrogen atom from glutamine's Δ place. As a consequence, the third nitrogen in the IMP is primarily extracted from the 5-007 role of glutamine. Similarly, during the synthesis of uridine monophosphate (UMP), a precursor of pyrimidine, glutamine leads to both Δ and Δ nitrogen atoms. However, the addition of aspartate 5-007 nitrogen is followed by three aspartate carbon atoms for the creation of an orotate chain. Since the carbon backbone of aspartate is produced from the tricarboxylic acid (TCA) process, and is replenished by glutamine-related 5-007-ketoglutarate, glutamine is also the main source of carbon atoms for UMP.

Second, glutamine can control the TCA process and the production of ATP. One explanation for cancer cells to depend on high amounts of exogenous glutamine is that glutamine may be used to drive the TCA process by 5-007-ketoglutarate to enable for more oxidation. Glutamine depletion has been shown to increased the NADH / NAD+ ratio, which decreases oxygen intake and ATP production. Therefore, in addition to the refilling of the TCA cycle intermediates for biosynthesis, the continuous oxidation of glutamine-derived 5-007-ketoglutarate via the TCA process often offers a source of energy.

Fourth, glutamine stimulates glutathione biosynthesis and

NADPH production to reduce oxidative stress. Glutamine facilitates the biosynthesis of glutathione, the main cell antioxidant, by at least two pathways.

As de novo biosynthesis of glutathione includes glutamate, cysteine and glycine, glutamine-derived glutamate is thus a direct substrate of glutathione biosynthesis. In addition, intracellular cysteine is primarily formed by the reduction of cystine, which is absorbed into cells at the cost of the export of glutamate via the xCT transporter. This is for the same purpose that xCT-positive triple-negative breast cancer cells are vulnerable to glutamine deficiency owing to inability to sustain intracellular cysteine for glutathione development and antioxidant protection. In addition, glutamine may contribute to the redox balance via the development of NADPH. However, glutamine does not act as a base in this case. Instead, it requires the catabolism of glutamine into the TCA process to create aspartate, which is shuttled through the cytosol and eventually transformed to oxaloacetate, malate and pyruvate.

The final stage of these reactions is catalyzed by the malic enzyme 1 (ME1) which passes electrons to NADP+ to generate NADPH. Along this axis, glutamine-dependent redox regulation produces potential weaknesses in KRAS-driven lung cancers with KEAP1 mutations that trigger the NRF2 pathway to alleviate oxidative stress.

Non-Biosynthetic Role of Glutamine

The fact that glutamine has been a key factor in the synthesis of amino acids in cancer can also be due to its non-biosynthetic role. It has been shown that glutamine-derived metabolites not only have precursors for macromolecules, but also serve as substrates or co-factors for the modulation of cellular processes. A convincing example is glutamine-derived 5-007-ketoglutarate, which is used as a co-substrate for a group of dioxygenase enzymes to mediate DNA and histone demethylation. Glutamine deficiency in the central nucleus of tumor tissues has been reported to lead to histone hypermethylation in the melanoma model by means of a melanoma-dependent 5-007-ketoglutarate system.

As a consequence of global histone hypermethylation, gene expression was changed, contributing to dedifferentiation and tolerance to the BRAF inhibitor in the xenograft mouse model. More work with other tumor models that hijack epigenetic machinery for progression is anticipated to provide a deeper view of the effect of glutamine supply on gene expression during tumor development or exposure to chemo-agents. Glutamine-derived 5-007-ketoglutarate has also been shown to regulate gene expression via histone and DNA demethylation in murine embryonic stem (ES) cells, T lymphocytes and macrophages.

Broad knowledge of the signal aspect that controls the accessibility of glutamine or catabolism to provide global regulation of gene expression in both tumor and immune cells should open up new possibilities to uncover the complexities of the tumor system in order to promote the creation of more successful immunotherapy.

Glutamine is also a beneficial growth-promoting signalling regulator. The best described glutamine-activated signaling is the mammalian target of rapamycin complex 1 (mTORC1), it was first stated that intracellular glutamine may be used as a counter-ion for the exchange of extracellular essential amino acids (EAAs) that are crucial to mTORC1 activation and mTORC1-dependent cell development. Later, biochemical analyzes performed in mammalian cells and yeast have shown that glutamine can directly activate mTORC1, but independently of Rag GTPase necessary for leucine-dependent mTORC1 activation. In fact, glutamine-derived 5-007-ketoglutarate is involved in the recruitment of mTORC1 to the lysosome for its activation. Recent studies have shown that glutamine deficiency can inhibit the aggregation of MYC protein and MYC-dependent transcription of genes in colorectal cancer. While the process has yet to be elucidated, it includes the synthesis and management of glutamine-dependent adenosine via the 3′ UTR of MYC mRNA. Because the MYC-dependent reprogramming of glutamine metabolism is well established[34,35], this research shows the reciprocal modulation between MYC and glutamine metabolism, which can have a significant effect on the comprehension of the interplay between n.

Glutamine Starvation: An Experimental Condition or Pathophysiological Stress

Glutamine deficiency problems were first called to the attention of nutritionists who found that plasma glutamine rates decreased dramatically during severe injury. Similar symptoms were subsequently identified in several other neurological disorders, frequently correlated in elevated catabolic behavior to account for the lack of circulating glutamine. Of starters, muscle protein catabolism is used to sustain the concentration of plasma glutamine at a lower level during long-term fasting. For cancer cases, the accumulation of serum glutamine is therefore reduced. Tumor-associated symptoms, such as cachexia, were believed to be the result of decreased amounts of amino acids in circulation. As a consequence, glutamine intake in the diet has been found to minimize muscle loss and improve immune function in certain cancer patients undergoing chemotherapy.

In consideration of the assumption that cancer cells enhance the consumption of glutamine to promote biosynthesis, the reported decrease in the concentration of glutamine in the bloodstream of cancer patients indicates that glutamine restriction increasing occur throughout tumor development. Yes, the amounts of glutamine in tumor tissues or body fluids surrounding tumor tissues have been shown to be smaller than usual tissues or plasma. In comparison, recent research shows that glutamine has been more reduced in the center of xenograft tumors, also inside the same tumor tissue, relative to the perimeter of the tumors. This finding is compatible with the idea that insufficient vascular nutrient supply remains a obstacle to internal tumor mass accumulation. As a consequence, comprehensive attempts have lately been made to clarify the various pathways utilized by tumor cells to respond to the restriction of glutamine for further development. Such pathways include signaling-mediated decision on cell fate, proteolytic scavenging, improved de novo biosynthesis of glutamine, and rewiring the usage of certain nutrients.

Influence of Other Amino Acids on Glutamine Starvation

Interested studies conducted over the last five years indicate that accessibility to certain nutrients, especially NEAAs, may have a profound impact on the response of tumor cells to glutamine starvation. Asparagine, aspartate and arginine demonstrate the ability to protect tumor cells from glutamine starvation or block glutamine catabolism, while cystine uptake increases cell sensitivity to such disturbances. In the next few sections, we will discuss the impact of each of these findings on the understanding of the metabolism of glutamine and its potential therapeutic applications in cancer.

Asparagine

Asparagine, an NEAA that can be synthesized de novo from glutamine, has been found to be capable of suppressing glutamine-depletion-induced apoptosis in brain tumor cells. Since all brain tumor cells studied were preserved in a normal DMEM medium comprising 6 mM of glutamine but without five NEAAs, including alanine, proline, glutamate, aspartate and asparagine, the authors performed a detailed metabolomic study to measure intracellular metabolites following glutamine depletion in the presence or absence of extracellular asparagine supplementation. Of interest, asparagine supplementation does not rescue the levels of the other four NEAAs (Ala, Pro, Glu and Asp) or any intermediate TCA cycle, both of which are significantly reduced by depletion of glutamine.

This paper highlights the importance of other nutrients in modulating the response of tumor cells to glutamine starvation and also raises an important question as to what is the most critical glutamine-derived metabolite for tumor cells to survive glutamine starvation. Mechanically, asparagine rescues cell survival at least partially by inhibiting endoplasmic reticulum (ER) stress caused by glutamine starvation. Later, the same group showed that the effect of asparagine on cell adaptation to glutamine starvation is generalizable in multiple tumor types.

In several epithelial breast tumor lines, asparagine has been shown to even rescue the spread defect during glutamine starvation without restoring other intermediate NEAAs and TCA cycles at steady-state levels. In this study, the authors have shown that asparagine can rescue global protein synthesis that is disrupted by glutamine starvation, and this process is facilitated by enhanced post-transcriptional expression of glutamine synthetase (GLUL) in an asparagine-dependent manner.

These two works suggest that most glutamine-dependent biosynthetic activities will proceed, with the exception of asparagine development, when exogenous glutamine is not present. Interestingly, the research performed in vasculature-forming endothelial cells and Kaposi's sarcoma-associated herpesvirus (KSHV)-transformed fibroblast cells revealed a related influence of asparagine to promote cell survival and proliferation following depletion of glutamine.

Importantly, asparagine can recover glutamine-depletion-induced growth defect in breast tumor cells at rates within the physiological range (25~100 µM). Throughout this level of concentrations, none of the other NEAAs is capable of retrieving the distribution. In addition, the introduction of catalytically active asparaginase, an enzyme that breaks down asparagine, from lower vertebrates to mammalian cells, prevents asparagine from rescuing glutamine starvation at physiological concentrations. As putative human asparaginase displays limited asparaginase activity, the writers focus on the evolutionary pressure to induce selective loss of function in mammalian cells as a way of maintaining intracellular asparagine to mediate cell tolerance to pathophysiological shifts in environmental glutamine rates

In addition, as with glutamine, intracellular asparagine was also found to be capable of acting as a counter ion for the exchange of extracellular EAAs for the maintenance of mTORC1 activity. Supplementation of asparagine in a DMEM medium that does not regularly contain asparagine-maintain mTORC1 activity, which is otherwise suppressed by deprivation of glutamine. It remains to be established if the restoration of mTORC1 function by asparagine supplementation plays a role in the growth / survival of tumor cells during glutamine starvation.

Aspartate and Arginine

In addition to asparagine, two recent papers have shown that aspartate, another NEAA that can be synthesized from glutamine-derived carbon and nitrogen atoms, plays a critical role in the adaptation of tumor cells to glutamine starvation or inhibit glutamine catabolism have shown that aspartate absorption through its SLC1A3 cell surface transporter can help tumor cell proliferation under glutamine.

Tumor suppressor is necessary for transcriptional induction of SLC1A3 following depletion of glutamine. In another independent review, it has been shown that release of aspartate from mitochondria to cytosol plays a critical role in mediating tumor cell survival and proliferation in low glutamine environments or after pharmacological inhibition of glutamine, a main enzyme for glutamine catabolism and further use. This transfer of mitochondrial aspartate to cytosol is regulated by the mitochondrial aspartate-glutamate carrier 1 (AGC1) and the genetic repression of AGC1 inhibits the development of xenograft tumors when the glutaminase inhibitor is used. Mechanically, both studies have shown that aspartate is a crucial precursor to nucleotide biosynthesis, but dependence on aspartate to help TCA cycle intermediates and other NEAAs is not needed for cell growth during inhibition of glutaminease.

Arginine has recently been shown to support the adaptation of tumor cells to glutamine starvation. Glutamine deprivation has been shown to induce the expression of arginine transporter SLC7A3 on the cell surface in a-dependent manner to facilitate the uptake of arginine. As a consequence, intracellular arginine aggregation promotes mTORC1 activation and cell growth / proliferation. For note, arginine does not add to the TCA process by transforming ornithine to glutamate or fumarate during the urea stage. More research is needed that it will help the biosynthesis of other macromolecules during glutamine starvation.

Cystine

Cystine, as compared to asparagine, aspartate and arginine, was found to improve the ability of the tumor cells to suppress glutaminase when complemented above physiological levels in the tissue culture medium. Because cystine absorption through the xCT transporter uses glutamate as a counter ion in exchange, it was proposed that the exchange of cystine /

glutamate generates dependency on glutamine to sustain glutamine deamination and glutamate output. Imports of cystine as a central component of glutamine / glutamate-dependent antioxidant protection have been recorded of value. These research together may indicate that accurate regulation of the use of glutamine is required for controlled tumor development, particularly when the supply of exogenous glutamine is compromised. Tumor cells depend on glutamine-derived glutamate for the exchange of cystine, which is the main source of intracellular cysteine, NEAA for protein synthesis and for the development of glutathione; on the other hand, excessive cystine absorption can induce glutamate depletion, preventing more use of cystine via the TCA process or transamination.

What Is the Critical Limiting Metabolite during Glutamine Starvation

Both of the above findings indicate the presence of a systematic system to mediate the sensitivity of tumor cells to the restriction of glutamine. However, the fact that more than one amino acid can alter the response of tumor cells to glutamine starvation or its catabolic inhibition poses a challenge to the efficacy of targeting the metabolism of glutamine in cancer. One interesting problem that might emerge is why tumor cells prefer specific amino acids to modulate their dependency on exogenous glutamine. The simplest answer is that there is a difference in the inherent properties of tumor cells. This specificity can be determined by tumor origin, oncogene / tumor suppression status, and the microenvironment of the tumor. For example, it can be expected that tumors with p53 lack of function may not be able to respond to glutamine starvation due to aspartate or arginine uptake. Further work is required to establish complementary approaches that can be coupled to control the synthesis of glutamine in cancer.

Another approach to address the abundance of certain amino acids that enable the tolerance of tumor cells that impaired glutamine metabolism is to identify the most important restricting metabolite. The fact that asparagine alone is capable of saving cell proliferation without restoring the intermediate TCA cycle and other glutamine-derived NEAAs following the depletion of glutamine is a compelling example. In this review, the authors demonstrate that supplementation of exogenous glutamine at 0.1 mM can not promote cell proliferation as well as the same concentration of asparagine.

Because cell proliferation needs both glutamine and asparagine, this finding indicates that asparagine biosynthesis, but not glutamine itself, is a limiting factor for epithelial breast tumor cells to proliferate when exogenous glutamine is small. It should be remembered that asparagine was also observed to be lower in tumor tissues relative to usual surrounding tissues. Asparagine was observed to be about 30 μM in the center of xenografted tumor tissues, which is 25% of the asparagine amounts in the periphery of the same tumor tissues. At this concentration, asparagine is likely to be sufficient to support protein synthesis to allow limited amounts of glutamine to be used for other biosynthetic reactions.

However, one may doubt why tumor cells can not easily use glutamine-derived carbon and nitrogen to synthesize asparagine through asparagine synthetase (ASNS), an enzyme that is highly expressed in solid tumor cells, unless glutamine itself is restricting. A new study reveals that the relative biosynthetic energy rate of asparagine is the largest of the nine NEAAs (Asn, Asp, Gln, Ser, Arg, Pro, Glu, Ala, Gly) that are synthesized from glycolysis and the TCA-derived carbon source in humans.

This is possibly due to the high energy expense of sustaining the glucose carbon flow into the TCA process to produce glutamate, glutamine and aspartate while exogenous glutamine is not available. We may assume that while tumor cells produce high rates of ASNS, they are unable to afford sufficient energy for the development of asparagine. In particular, glutamine itself is necessary for protein synthesis. In this respect, asparagine promotes glutamine synthesis de novo through post transcription activation of glutamine synthetase (GLUL) during glutamine starvation.

Key Variants Impacting the Definition of Critical Limiting Metabolite

Defining the essential restricting metabolite in each sense would not only elucidate the fundamental connection between the biochemistry of glutamine metabolism and its biological functions, but can also include novel metabolic targets that can be blocked to improve the effectiveness of targeting glutamine metabolism in cancer. However, many variables need to be addressed rigorously in order to determine the essential restricting metabolite.

First, the amino acid concentration of the tissue culture

medium determines the forms of deprivation. When setting Dulbecco's modified Eagle medium (DMEM), which does not contain exogenous asparagine and aspartate, glutamine deprivation is expected to cause intracellular depletion of at least these three amino acids. In comparison, Medium 199 contains all NEAAs with the exception of asparagine, and so the deficiency of glutamine can cause the depletion of glutamine and asparagine, but not aspartate. Likewise, in comparison to both NEAAs, glutamine deficiency will only deplete glutamine itself until aspartate intake is prevented. In this situation, the absorption of excess aspartate via its cell surface transporter can not only rescue aspartate-dependent nucleotide and protein synthesis, but can also enable the re-uptake of TCA cycle intermediates to trigger de novo biosynthesis of glutamine.

Second, glutamine deficiency and inhibition of glutamine can identify various types of essential restricting metabolites. Under laboratory settings where exogenous glutamine is depleted or decreased to a low amount, it may be concluded that all glutamine-dependent cellular pathways are affected. Nevertheless, glutamine inhibition is predicted to prevent the conversion of glutamine to glutamate and its further use in the TCA process, NEAA development and nucleotide biosynthesis. In this environment, intracellular glutamine itself and any glutamine-dependent growth / survival signaling is not supposed to be reduced.

The fact that exogenous aspartate rescues glutaminase inhibition by nucleotide synthesis but not by the TCA cycle and other NEAAs indicates that such metabolic activities that continue, possibly through using other carbon sources in the tissue culture medium, it should be remembered that glutamine is also an indispensable nitrogen source for nucleotide biosynthesis independently of aspartate. The fact that glutamine itself is unrestricted following inhibition of glutamine may clarify why these cells do not need exogenous aspartate to sustain the TCA cycle, a required process for de novo biosynthesis of glutamine.

Third, the essential limiting metabolite important for cell proliferation and survival that vary with respect to the restriction of glutamine. Because cell proliferation involves accumulation of biomass, it can be predicted that when a single amino acid will rescue cell proliferation during glutamine deficiency or inhibition of glutamine, biosynthesis of all macromolecules will be able to start.

Throughout this environment, tumor cells must maintain their capacity to accumulate an sufficient amount of amino acids, like asparagine, aspartate, glutamate and glutamine for protein synthesis. In addition, each of these amino acids must be obtained at rates necessary to enable the biosynthesis of certain macromolecule precursors. For example, aspartate and glutamine are indispensable precursors for the biosynthesis of nucleotides. However, where a single amino acid can only rescue a survival defect, such as arginine, macromolecule biosynthesis is not necessary. Indeed, the most critical limiting metabolites for cell survival under different types of metabolic stress remain elusive. However, improvements in signalling mechanisms including nutrient processing, stress reaction and apoptosis are believed to be key players.

Complexity of Glutamine Starvation in Tumors In Vivo

Like in vitro cell culture studies in which we can specifically monitor the volume of nutrient in tissue culture material, the abundance of nutrients in the tumor setting fluctuates. By addition, tumors with low nutritional availability have a greater risk of suffering from glutamine malnutrition, as well as of participating by adaptive processes to relieve stress. Also with an adequate systemic supply, the production of glutamine in the circulation and body fluids is many times smaller relative to other tissue culture outlets.

At the other side, unlike in vitro studies in which tumor cells are sometimes exposed to intense depletion of glutamine, the tension induced by the restriction of glutamine in in vivo tumor cells may be offset to some degree by a low rate of continuous supply. In order to assess the dependency of tumor cells on exogenous glutamine at nutritional status similar to physiological levels, a new formula incorporating nutrients was established at concentrations comparable to the human serum. Glioma cells may develop in this medium without exogenous glutamine. In this setting, glutamine needed for cell growth can be synthesized de novo by GLUL in glioma cells or astrocytes in the tumor area.

The capacity of glioma cells to receive glutamine from astrocytes tells us of the significance of certain cell forms co-existing in the microenvironment of the tumor. Models of ovarian cancer and prostate cancer have demonstrated that cancer-associated fibroblasts (CAFs) can synthesize glutamine de novo and secrete glutamine to promote tumor cell growth in a glutamine-limiting setting.

In comparison to stromal cells, macrophages in the tumor community may lead to the development of the tumor by glutamine synthesis. Macrophage polarization during glutamine malnutrition has been shown to support M2-like fate in a GLUL-dependent fashion, which promotes immunosuppression and tumor metastases. Blocking GLUL in macrophages preserved M1-like phenotype, facilitated cytotoxic T cell activity and blocked metastases.

Nonetheless, more research is needed if macrophages rely on glutamine biosynthesis to help their own macromolecule biosynthesis or glutamine-dependent signaling and gene expression. The availability of stroma-dependent nutrients is not restricted to glutamine. Within a prostate cancer model, stroma cells can synthesize and secrete asparagine for tumor cells to respond to a glutamine-limiting environment. This capacity to synthesize asparagine includes the activation of ASNS-dependent transcription factor 4 (ATF4) expression in stroma cells. However, it could be hypothesized that stroma cells use a process other than tumor cells for the production of glutamine, as de novo asparagine synthesis is not energetically desirable in the absence of exogenous glutamine.

In addition, recent research indicates that the exchange of glutamate / aspartate between tumor cells and stromal fibroblast cells is essential for the maintenance of tumor cell growth and stromal cell function. Whether this unusual reliance on the exchange of glutamate / aspartate illustrates the weakness of environmental glutamine remains to be understood

Therapeutic Implication

After the first mention of "glutamine dependency" in cancer

cells, the potential for controlling glutamine metabolism has been widely explored in pre-clinical models. Nevertheless, the presence of a number of adaptive mechanisms to mitigate stress induced by glutamine limitation plus a complicated tumor microenvironment can present functional challenges. Thanks to toxicity and lack of accuracy, most of the molecular regulators of glutamine synthesis and catabolism are only used as aid compounds.

The best-developed small molecule is CB-839, a potent mitochondrial glutaminase (GLS) receptor, and the only one widely used in clinical trials in cancer patients. Because GLS catalyzes the conversion of glutamine to glutamate, therapy is required to deplete intracellular glutamate and prevent its further usage in the TCA cycle, NEAA development and nucleotide biosynthesis.

Physiological responses to repression of glutamine are likely to be distinct from the suppression of glutamine in tumor cells. For mouse models of lung cancer and glioma, the entrance of glutamine-derived carbon into the TCA cycle is regulated for vivo, which coincides with CB-839 tolerance.

Such findings do not preclude the value of glutamine to help tumor development, but indicate that these tumors do not depend on glutamine-derived carbon to sustain the TCA cycle. Throughout this respect, the contribution of glutamine-derived nitrogen to tumor growth throughout vivo has not been measured, partially because most of these reactions do not depend on glutamine production. More research is required to decide if the increased dependency of some tumors on glutamine-derived carbon to sustain the TCA cycle is a decision taken by tumor cells or merely a result of a restricted availability of glutamine.

In any scenario, may we distinguish specific features in the tumor tissue of origin or the oncogene / tumor suppressor status correlated with their reliance on glutamine? As described earlier, the supply of glutamine in the tumor environment is always restricted. The ability of tumor cells to use both glutamine-derived carbon and other carbon sources to power the TCA cycle may represent metabolic plasticity depending on the availability of environmental nutrients.

Another distinction in stimulation of glutamine and lack of glutamine is the presence of other glutamine-converting enzymes that may substitute for the stimulation of glutamine. Those comprise enzymes in the biosynthesis of asparagine, nucleotide, NAD and glucosamine. Both such enzymes transfer the Δ nitrogen of glutamine to their substrates, thus producing glutamate as a by-product. It is still uncertain whether these pathways can compensate in some cases where inhibition of glutamine is not successful. In order to avoid the procurement of glutamine for clinical action that mimics the deficiency of glutamine, a recent study identified a small molecule receptor, V-9302, which blocks the activity of the glutamine transporter (ASCT2).

In this research, V-9302 inhibited the absorption of glutamine in a wide variety of solid tumor lines as well as in many xenograft tumor models, contributing to a profound defect in tumor cell growth and survival. However, ASCT2 is also used for the processing of certain amino acids, such as leucine, and V-9302 may also inhibit the absorption of leucine. It would be necessary to assess the possible toxicity of normal cells that may use ASCT2 for the import of amino acids. In addition, the analysis of ASCT2-dependency in various types or subtypes of tumors is important in order to guide the application of this new compound. In the future, investigating glutamine dependency in additional tumor models with more complex criteria at various stages of tumor development, including onset, systemic invasion, metastases, or chemotherapy reaction, should offer more insight into the therapeutic effects of recognizing the synthesis of glutamine in cancer under physiological conditions.

Because tumor cells may use certain amino acids to alleviate tension induced by glutamine deficiency or suppression of glutamine catabolism, the acquisition and synthesis of such amino acids should be viewed at least as a complementary strategy when targeting the synthesis of glutamine in cancer. For starters, exogenous asparagine is a resource restricting the growth of acute lymphoblastic leukemia (ALL) cells due to their failure to synthesize asparagine de novo.

As a consequence, L-asparaginase, a bacterial enzyme that can kill asparagine in the bloodstream, has been used to effectively treat pediatric ALL patients for decades. However, L-asparaginase is unlikely to be involved in the treatment of solid tumors owing to its failure to synthesize sufficiently asparagine. Yet integrating L-asparaginase with glutamine synthesis inhibitors can be a rational approach to improve the therapeutic result. Recent research has demonstrated that L-asparaginase alone can reduce the risk of breast cancer metastases to the lung without altering tumor development at the primary site.

Further analysis is needed if this finding represents a deficiency of glutamine in the lung or during the metastasis phase. Similar to L-asparaginase, arginine-depleting enzyme, arginine deiminase (ADI) is used in several clinical trials for solid tumors based on the finding that some forms of tumors suppress the production of arginine biosynthetic enzymes and are thus arginine auxotrophic. It is worth exploring if ADI can be paired with metabolic reduction of glutamine for improved clinical outcomes.

Given the increasingly growing awareness of the synthesis of glutamine and its complex biological roles in cancer, obstacles remain until this mechanism can be widely utilized in the care of cancer patients. Next, we need to identify different pathways to mediate the sensitivity of tumor cells to the restriction of glutamine. Tumor cells can respond to the restriction of glutamine via a number of pathways, representing the metabolic plasticity that can be chosen as a means of improved nutrient consumption during tumor development. The basic pathway selected by the tumor cell is the form or subtype of the tumor, the oncogene / tumor suppressor status, the location of the tumor and the level of tumor growth. Defining a particular adaptive function may not only make it possible to determine whether or not to target the metabolism of glutamine, but may also give insight into potential mechanisms that will need to be blocked together to improve the effectiveness of targeting the metabolism of glutamine. Second, because the existence of certain nutrients may have a significant impact on tumor cell reaction to glutamine restriction, it is important to identify the specific nutritional status in the tumor setting.

Apparently, the bulk of mass spectrometry (MS)-based nutrient quantification from primary tumor tissues does not discriminate between nutrient rates inside tumor cells or in the local tumor setting. In fact, an appropriate procedure must be created to isolate tumor cells, stromal cells and immune cells from the same tumor tissue in a timely manner for metabolic assessment. Third, we need to understand further the metabolic interaction between tumor cells and immune cells, such as T cells, when glutamine uptake or catabolism is compromised.

This has come to light that other glutamine-dependent cell roles have gone beyond cancer cells. Among T cells, the destruction of glutamine synthesis and catabolism has a significant impact on T cell differentiation and immune response.

Therefore, differential responses to the restriction of glutamine or glutamine-derived metabolites between tumor cells and T cells should ensure therapeutic approaches that suppress tumor growth while preserving the effector and cytotoxic role of T cells. In the future, it is our hope that facts will turn up and close the holes of our knowledge in these fields. By this point, we will no longer need to think about developing a "hungry beast" of starving glutamine cancer cells.

CPSIA information can be obtained
at www.ICGtesting.com
Printed in the USA
BVHW041515190321
602997BV00010B/537

9 781801 876445